The Bone-Building Solution

The Bone-Building Solution

By Sam Graci, Dr. Leticia Rao,
and Dr. Carolyn DeMarco

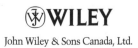

John Wiley & Sons Canada, Ltd.

National Library of Canada Cataloguing in Publication Data

Graci, Sam, 1946-
The bone-building solution / Sam Graci, Leticia Rao, Carolyn DeMarco

Includes bibliographical references and index.

ISBN-13: 978-0-470-83891-4

    1. Bones—Diseases—Prevention. 2. Women—Health and hygiene.
I. Rao, Leticia Gomez, 1939- II. Title.

RC931.O73G73 2006   616.7'105   C2006-902216-X

Production Credits:
Cover design: Natalia Burobina
Interior text design: Pat Loi
Printer: Printcrafters

John Wiley & Sons Canada, Ltd.
6045 Freemont Blvd.
Mississauga, Ontario
L5R 4J3

Printed in Canada

3 4 5 PC 10 09 08 07

Table of Contents

Acknowledgments

Dedicated to:
You, the reader, because you are willing to "upgrade" and revitalize your life.

Very special thanks to:
Stewart Brown for his enthusiasm that turned dreams into reality. A really true friend through thick and thin.

Karen Corley for her endless encouragement, boundless commitment and extremely talented, good-spirited editing of the manuscript. Purna Ma for her insights and exquisite scholarship. Elvira Clare for her right word, in the right place, at the right time, so many times. Mark Huthmacher for his unfailing encouragement. Dianne Fidler for her many days and nights at the computer. My brother, Joe Graci, for his generous and tireless research assistance that improved every chapter of this book.

Special thanks to:
Tara Stubensey, Janice Partington, Beth Potter, and Lisa Chisholm-Neal for their critical and welcomed editorial input. Dr. Alan Logan for his timely resourcefulness, thoughtful advice and willingness to share his knowledge of nutritional biochemistry.

Endless thanks to:

The exceptionally skilled and talented team from John Wiley & Sons Publishing: Robert Harris, General Manager, a very special kind of man; Jennifer Smith, Publisher, for her superb literary guidance; Valerie Ahwee, for her high-energy, highly-skilled and painstaking editing, as well as her invaluable knowledge and humor.

Leah Marie Fairbank, Editor, for her enthusiasm, skilled advice, diligent attention, and unrelenting dedication—who navigated the development of this book with courage and patient foresight.

Liz McCurdy and Pamela Vokey, Project Managers, for their superb talent and guidance and for embracing this project. Pat Loi for her amazing persistence in perfecting the interior design. Natalia Burobina and Ian Koo who helped conceive, design, and develop the front cover for this book. Meghan Brousseau, the talented Publicist; and so many others for their wonderful support in creatively shaping this book.

Part I

Factoring in the Bone-Building Solution— A Comprehensive Plan

CHAPTER 1

Dramatically Improve Your Bones, Joints, and Fluid Movements

In many ways this is the most exciting book I have written to date. My purpose is to provide you with optimal recommendations based on the latest persuasive, consistent, and breakthrough research in achieving better bone and joint health, strong structure, good posture, and fluid biomechanical movement for a lifetime.

The Bone-Building Solution presents a research-proven, radical new idea—the first comprehensive action plan that could alter the course of the common "silent epidemic" of stiff joints, aching bones, weak bone strength, poor tooth enamel, brittle nails, and osteoporosis (OP) in children, men, and women. Poor bone health is a concern not only for those in midlife and older. In fact, recent studies have shown that increasing numbers of younger people are affected by porous, weak bones, poor posture, and deteriorating tooth quality because of poor lifestyle choices.

Poor nutrition, a lack of proper exercise that promotes core strength and balanced equilibrium, and an inadequate supplement program are the leading causes of bone and joint-related disease. In medicine, however, old and long-used treatments are sometimes slow to change. The traditional approach of using drugs to treat men and women with OP not only covers up the symptoms without addressing the root cause, it can also cause significant suffering on its own while the disease progresses further. The most commonly prescribed bisphosphonate drug treatments do not address the true causes of porous, weak bones.

Nutritional deficiencies in our 206 bones and 143 joints occur long before they're evident on an X-ray or a standardized blood test. Bone-repair and bone-building capabilities are extremely sensitive to daily, erratic, suboptimal supplies of all-important vitamins, minerals, protein, and fats. Bone-building metabolism declines dramatically during times of nutrient deficiencies. When our diet and supplements restore vitamin, mineral, protein, and healthy fats, bone-repair and bone-building capabilities resume at full capacity.

As a nutritional and lifestyle researcher, I have great respect for conventional medicine and the many miracles it can perform. In fact, the step-by-step action plan in this book is well on the path to becoming the standard first line of prevention or treatment with many progressive doctors and health care providers.

THE BEST MEDICAL BONE BREAK-THROUGHS IN THE 21ST CENTURY

The information presented in this book is based on a rational interpretation of breakthrough scientific and medical research. This is the future that will allow you to stand tall, maintain a great range of comfortable motion, experience the ease of correct posture, and keep your teeth and nails strong—for every day of your life.

Typically, other books on bone health present one or two new ideas combined with a lot of old information. Instead, we provide a high density of new ideas on how to harness breakthrough research to offer you unprecedented health benefits.

There is always the potential to improve your personal bone health and fluid biomechanical movement. The distinguishing feature that makes us human is the constant search and awareness to understand the world around us—and to be courageous in making significant departures from the old status quo.

The most important principle of *The Bone-Building Solution* is an active exploration of new knowledge from multiple sources.

Ten breakthroughs you will master are:

- New insights into natural "molecular-targeted" bone-building therapeutics

- Newly available bone mineral density (BMD) diagnosis and treatment options elucidated by Dr. Carolyn DeMarco, M.D., emerging from today's scientific breakthroughs

- Surprising information revealing that doctor-endorsed DEXA bone scans do not give accurate or definitive information on the micro-architectural structure or strength of your 206 bones—misdiagnosis is common and subsequent widespread use of bisphosphonate medications may be fraught with errors

- Cutting-edge knowledge about your own personal condition and how to keep it humming at peak efficiency for the future

- How to determine where you are located in the progression of the age-related bone degenerative process and how to reverse it—now! You can decide for yourself what changes and fine-tuning you are willing to make with contemporary bone-repair and bone-building knowledge to transform your own health

- Revolutionary discoveries by University of Toronto clinical researcher Dr. Leticia Rao, Ph.D., on how our diet has the power to radically improve or impair our bone-building, bone-repair and bone health—and why!

- Dr. Alan C. Logan, N.D., of Harvard Medical School presents his most important discovery ever—"bone smart" fish oils—for perpetual upgraded bone-repair and bone-building

- The renowned Dr. John Berardi, Ph.D., of the University of Texas emphasizes that strong bones are usually attached to strong, well developed muscles—our bones, in fact, weaken and thin at about the same rate as our muscles atrophy. Exercising for healthy muscle mass indicates that we are putting stress on the bones, and our bones grow stronger in response to the mechanical stress (called loading) we put on them

- All researchers agree that adequate calcium is absolutely essential for development, repair, and maintenance of bone health—the question, however, is just what comprises an adequate calcium intake—you may be surprised by what Dr. Leticia Rao's clinical research reveals

- Because of their amazing complexity, our bones and joints have remained shrouded in mystery as researchers were not exactly sure how to easily repair their mechanical hardware from daily wear-and-tear—until now.

Today, mastering your bone destiny is a lot easier than you might think.

My Mother's Story

My mother's story is pretty typical of many people. Despite her initial misgivings, she was willing to undertake the necessary steps to overcome her worsening symptoms of weak, aching bones, stiff joints, brittle nails, and failing tooth enamel. Her hair lustre and skin quality were also deteriorating. I had her begin a daily walking program in the fresh air and sunshine. She began to eat more salads, color-coded vegetables, deep-pigmented berries, seasonal fruit, and lean protein. She reduced stress with effective prayer and meditation. She also used a bone-building supplement to overcome nutritional inconsistencies and to reduce inflammation, which is one of the hallmarks of aging and chronic disease.

These effective lifestyle changes gave her surprising benefits in 21 days—and a more positive mental outlook. Your taste buds have a memory of about 21 days, and in that time Mama's taste preferences changed. After your taste buds adjust, your desire for sugary, salty, fatty, or heavy foods will diminish dramatically.

She was willing to undertake the necessary steps and became more enthusiastic as her energy soared. Her skin became more supple and toned, and therefore wrinkles disappeared. Her brittle nails strengthened, and her bone and tooth strength improved progressively. Her range of fluid movement increased by 60 percent.

Remarkably so, my mother, at 68 years of age, lost 25 lbs. And, while this book's bone-building strategy doesn't focus on weight loss, you also, if necessary, will naturally lose weight as you follow the practical, easy to follow, step-by-step action plan in this book.

My motivation for writing this book is to spare you or a loved one the stiffness, pain, stooped posture, downtime, and loss of critical bone mass my mother experienced unnecessarily.

BECOME A MASTER OF LIFE: DEVELOP A NEW KIND OF AWARENESS

Every life is a remarkable story ready to be told. Biochemical processes, which have been naturally selected in the "divine blueprint" to protect us from disease and premature aging, become increasingly derailed in most people after the age of 34. You need to have knowledge. Knowledge is power when it comes to daily restoring, renewing, rejuvenating, and reinvigorating your 100 trillion faithful cells.

Become part of a new generation of men and women willing to take charge of their own health destiny. The effort will reward you with immediate frequent-flyer miles, including heightened brainpower, increased emotional stability, and bone-building upgrades. These are worthwhile and achievable goals for everyone. There is really no other effective alternative.

THE "SANDWICH GENERATION"

In the following pages I will explore with you the enormous wealth of new research discoveries and practical information to guide you in the care and maintenance of your bones, stature, posture, movement, teeth, nails, and, surprisingly, your heart. We all would like lifetime immunity from disease and illness, and we are slowly closing in on that goal. But we need to help ourselves and not allow our health to become unhinged by our very own eating habits, sleep deprivation, lack of exercise, lack of proper supplementation, and accumulated acute stress load.

We especially need to get the message of healthy eating and exercise out to our children and teens, as the lifestyle choices they make now will affect their bone-building and overall health for a lifetime. It is estimated that 60 percent of North Americans are overweight or obese, including 26 percent of children ages six to 19.

Many of us between the ages of 35 and 65 are part of the so-called "sandwich generation." You may be caring for both children who are very young, teenagers, or in their twenties or thirties, and parents or a spouse who are beginning to experience serious health conditions. It is imperative that you take especially good care of your precious well-being and health, and bone-building functions. Your decisions have implications for all those lives you are privileged to touch in your lifetime. This is the type of thinking that will push bone-building to its next frontier.

DON'T BE LOST IN TRANSLATION: SENSE AND SENSITIVITY

"Survival of the fittest" was a proper adaptation response for our ancient biological ancestors to survive and flourish. However, to survive and flourish well today, we must adapt by a new rule of the road: "Survival of the wisest." The ancient mystery of how bone-building works and how we can make it work even better, particularly in the second half of our lives, is yielding to twenty-first-century research and knowledge.

There is a tremendous difference between information, understanding, and wisdom. Today we've gained enormous understanding of our physical world through a bounty of information, but we've lost sight of the wisdom of how we naturally fit into the world.

We used to know better. We've selfishly manipulated the rules and we feel unfulfilled because we have lost faith in our own innate wisdom—and it just might be time to get it back!

> *"When faced with the choice between changing and proving there's no need to do so, most people get busy on the proof."*
>
> —John Kenneth Galbraith

SAY GOODBYE TO ACHING BONES, SORE JOINTS, AND POOR POSTURE

The Bone-Building Solution offers hope and a practical plan for achieving and maintaining vibrant bone health. It is a comprehensive, easy-to-follow action plan that supports your 206 different bones and 143 different joints at their genetic roots. Today, you can ramp up your bone-repair and bone-building systems while dramatically improving your body's repair functions, stamina, endurance, good mood, bones, joints, and memory with a more youthful, radiant, healthy stature.

This information is not only reaching you but also your physician. There are a growing number of physicians who are specializing in these new medical breakthroughs and successfully implementing them with their patients. I will be introducing you to one such progressive and dedicated physician, Dr. Carolyn DeMarco, M.D., who contributes chapters 11 and 12 in this book.

Gone are the days when a few mysterious, elite researchers corresponded only among themselves. Years ago research findings were confined to scientific circles; all this was hidden from us. But today you need to keep informed and become part of the nutritional debate because your lifelong health is at stake.

To prove the point, when the *Journal of the American Medical Association* (*JAMA*) and *The New England Journal of Medicine* were launched in the nineteenth century, they did not have a publicity department to inform the public. Since 2004, the *JAMA* spends $1 million U.S. annually on its media and communication program to keep the public informed and updated, says the editor, Catherine DeAngelis, M.D.

In the Product Resources section at the back of this book you will find a list of 10 excellent monthly newsletters to keep you informed and updated.

A small number of dedicated medical scientists, who do the actual up-and-coming research, are now willing to reach out to the public. They specialize in perfecting new medical breakthrough solutions. I will be introducing you to a progressive and extremely dedicated husband-and-wife research team. One is Dr. Leticia Rao, Ph.D., Director of the Calcium Research Lab, St. Michael's Hospital, University of Toronto, Faculty of Medicine, who will, for the first time, directly present to you the results of her innovative bone-building research. She has contributed Chapter 13, "Clinical Breakthroughs in Bone-Building Research," to this book. I will also introduce you to the highly regarded and renowned nutritional researcher, Professor Emeritus Dr. Venket A. Rao, Ph.D., Department of Nutritional Sciences, University of Toronto, Faculty of Medicine.

Their innovative research and groundbreaking scientific nutritional solutions are now accessible to you and of enormous interest to a wide range of people who are looking for clearer answers, especially for maintaining superior bone health, which dictates the quality of your skeletal structure, stature, biomechanical movements, and physical appearance.

We collected an unprecedented 12,000 recent scientific studies from peer-reviewed journals to support the step-by-step, easy-to-follow, comprehensive bone-building solutions presented in this book, which is very important to me as a nutritional and lifestyle researcher. I have spent three full years talking with world-renowned bone-building researchers to ensure that this book contains the best and most encouraging information to sustain and enhance your well-being. It is a fresh "open window" to new, dramatic, scientific breakthroughs that will enable you to keep your bone structure healthy and strong for a lifetime.

The likelihood of getting osteoporosis depends on the amount of bone density achieved at peak growth, age 24, then both the rate and duration of bone loss. Proper nutrition, supplementation, and exercise in childhood is imperative for proper bone growth—but it is never too late to make a difference.

The literal Greek translation of the word "osteoporosis" is *osteo* (the bone), *poro* (is becoming porous), *sis* (and inflamed). Over time, unfortunately, osteoporosis can cause the loss and erosion of bone structure, strength, and function of our bones and joints in both men and women. The tiny fractions of cellular damage in bones that are not repaired daily accumulate over the years and eventually cause chronic structural, stature, posture, and mobility disorders and diseases. Nowhere is the damage more tragic than in the loss of our fluid biomechanical movement and independence in later life.

Each year about 2.5 million North American men and women will suffer a broken bone as a result of deterioration of bone strength. At no other time in our history have weak, porous, aching, stiff bones affected more people aged 25 and older than it does today. Over the last 20 years we have heard the constant message that weak bones result from inadequate calcium intake. Well, calcium alone is not the answer to our osteoporosis epidemic.

Not only does this book correct many misconceptions, it provides, in Chapter 10, five easy-to-follow steps that children, teens, women, and men can use daily to create superior bone structure, function, and health throughout their lifetime.

In the field of medicine, there is always a tug-of-war between maintaining the status quo of old, long-used treatments and accepting new scientific breakthroughs. In the end, our diligent research has allowed good science to win out and dramatic new scientific breakthrough solutions to replace the old. And that is where this book begins.

CHAPTER 2

New Hope for Bone-Building

Surprisingly, there is a clear cause and effect relationship between your diet and lifestyle, and your bone, brain and heart health, teeth and nails. Consequently, you can immediately apply the information in this new, groundbreaking book and take charge of your own bone and heart health. Make a few simple changes in your life and reap incredible benefits that you can see and feel in just a few days.

While this book offers promise of a new approach to bone health, it also opens the door to taking greater personal responsibility for your own well-being. *The Bone-Building Solution* differs from any other book on bone health in that it deals with bones, posture, structure, and biomechanical movement at their genetic roots with a step-by-step, comprehensive action plan to ramp up genetic repair systems with each of your 206 bones and within each of your 100 trillion cells. Healthy bones, healthy life, healthy you! This is the bone-building breakthrough solution!

The new millennium is ushering in unprecedented scientific and medical advances in bone-building research. A super-critical team of synergistic micronutrient

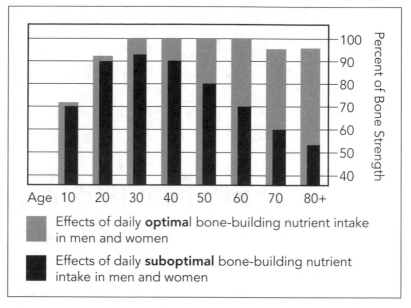

Figure 2.1: Optimal Bone Nutrient Intake—the Bone-Building Solution

(trace element) compounds has emerged from solid scientific research. These micronutrient compounds have been proven to both rejuvenate and turn "on" biological switches that quickly improve your internal bone-building functions, mobility, and posture all life long.

THE MIRACLE AND MARVEL OF STANDING TALL

The human body is a mechanical miracle and marvel with 206 different bones and 143 different joints that keep us erect, hold our structure, and enable us to stand and move. They also act as protectors, levers, shock absorbers, and hinges. Our head, jaw, teeth, neck, shoulders, back, vertebrae, ribs, arms, elbows, wrists, hands, fingers, hips, legs, knees, ankles, heels, feet, and toes perform thousands of motions that successfully propel us through a day.

Daily, these mechanical marvels need:

1. smart lifestyle choices
2. an optimal intake of bone-building nutrients
3. healthy bone-building metabolic exercise, and
4. food-based, "molecular-targeted" bone-building supplementation,

so that each and every bone can be strong and never crumble, grind, or stick in your lifetime.

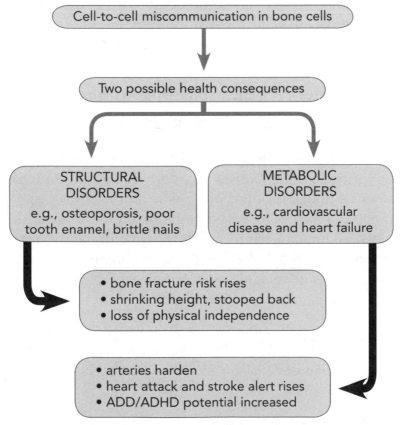

Figure 2.2: Daily Suboptimal Intake of Bone-Building Micronutrients and the Health Consequences

WHEN BONES AND POSTURE GO BAD

Our structure, posture, movements, balance, and appearance are the coordinated expression of healthy bones and joints. Most of us take them for granted; we are completely unaware of their marvel until something goes drastically wrong.

This book will focus on maintaining healthy bones; a firm but flexible structure; an attractive posture; good, radiant teeth; and strong clear nails. "Osteoporosis is inevitable after age 34," your doctor may tell you, "since everyone your age has some degree of it." But in fact, osteoporosis usually starts in both men and women in their twenties or even earlier, often many years before a person first notices symptoms.

WHAT ARE OSTEOPOROSIS AND OSTEOPENIA?

Osteoporosis is not a degenerative, inflammatory ailment just of the elderly. Nor is an overly accelerated break-down of your precious bone tissue an inevitable aspect of aging. Osteoporosis is a generalized disorder of the bones in our skeleton in which the quantity and quality of bone tissue is reduced and the micro-architecture of the bone makes it weak and susceptible to breaking, given even minimal amounts of trauma.

> The actual result of osteoporosis can be viewed as skeletal and bone failure, similar to heart failure, blood pressure failure, hearing failure, and vision failure after years of wear-and-tear.

There is no research evidence that bone loss is associated with pain or any other symptoms. According to Dr. Leticia Rao, Ph.D., Director of the Calcium Research Lab, St. Michael's Hospital, University of Toronto, Faculty of Medicine, "there are no symptoms of osteoporosis per se, only the consequences: fractures and associated chronic pain, deformity, and the unfortunate disability."

Osteopenia means that you have had some bone density and bone strength loss, but not a lot. It could be a forerunner or warning sign of future osteoporosis with further bone loss and fractures due to bone loss.

Some people can live a lifetime with osteopenia or osteoporosis and never have a bone fracture, whereas others will never develop severe osteoporosis but may break a bone. Having osteoporosis does not mean that you will inevitably suffer a fracture; however, nor does having normal or osteopenic bone density mean that you are completely risk free.

MYTH ONE: MY BONES JUST NEED MORE CALCIUM: MAKING SENSE OF THE CALCIUM AND VITAMIN D DEBATE

Years of conventional medical wisdom has suggested that we supplement with calcium and vitamin D to ensure that our bone-repair and bone-building systems will operate at optimum for a lifetime.

However, when the Women's Health Initiative published an influential study in the *New England Journal of Medicine*, questions were raised both about the study and about the benefits of taking supplements to prevent osteoporosis. "As I read and re-read them, the findings of the Women's Health Initiative on bone-building border on meaningless," wrote Jane E. Brody in the March 14, 2006 edition of *The New York Times* newspaper. Nearly two-thirds of the women in the placebo group had high intakes of calcium and vitamin D from diet alone, and many of those assigned to take the real calcium and vitamin D supplement failed to take them faithfully.

Did the women in the test group fully report their dietary habits? Self-reports of dietary intake are notoriously inaccurate. When the final results showed little difference between bone fracture risk of those taking a low-dose calcium and vitamin D supplement, many scientists blamed the poor study design. "It was a disappointment that the study was not better designed," says Joan Lappe, professor of medicine at the Osteoporosis Research Center at Creighton University. But to the average North American, the WHI study seemed like just one more example of nutritional scientists unable to make up their minds.

However, it did become clear that those women who took the assigned supplements at least 80 percent of the time experienced a 29 percent reduction in the risk of hip fractures during the seven-year study. That's positive!

In addition, a report published in the April 24, 2006 issue of the American Medical Association journal *Archives of Internal Medicine* concluded that bone-building supplements *are* an effective way to help prevent bone fractures in people who take them regularly. As it turns out, our most up-to-date research verifies that calcium is critical to bone density and bone strength, but as research scientists are learning, it just cannot work well all by itself.

Calcium as Part of a Synergistic, Bone-Building Team

Calcium, on its own, cannot reach the bone target bull's-eye. For example, bones require adequate protein daily to form the basic framework or scaffolding for bone-building. Healthy bones also require a daily mix of synergistic micronutrients, such as the following:

Vitamin K, known to be essential for blood clotting, encourages the maintenance of bones by signaling for structural proteins to be made while skillfully blocking proteins that help to break down bone. Vitamin K guides calcium into our 206 bones and keeps it out of soft tissue such as our brain, heart, and arteries where it can harden.

Silicon, often overlooked, is an abundant trace mineral in nature that is proving to be an essential ingredient for targeting stronger bones and may boost the benefits of calcium and bone calcification. Strontium is a mineral found along with calcium in most foods and required for normal development and health of the skeletal system.

We used to think that boron was useful only as a food preservative in the form of boric acid. By the 1970s it became clear that in people consuming small amounts of boron, their metabolism of calcium and magnesium improved. After taking boron supplements for eight days, the blood levels of bone-building estrogen and testosterone nearly doubled. Inadequate levels of the essential trace mineral copper have been associated with poor bone quality and osteoporosis.

Zinc is a heavy hitter when it comes to bone health and is a cofactor (that is, one of several elements that are required to work together for effective bone-building) in more than 200 enzyme reactions. Vitamin B12 (cobala-min), vitamin B9 (folic acid or folate), and vitamin B6 (pyridoxine) are water-soluble vitamins that produce hydrochloric acid in the stomach (so calcium and foods dissolve). These compounds are essential to bone health and calcium absorption. And the new kid on the block, lycopene (the red antioxidant carotenoid), which is found in tomatoes, pink grapefruit, red berries, and beets, helps bones stay strong and disease free.

Recently scientists have rallied around another new research breakthrough that fish oils rich in the essential fatty acids eicosapentaenoic acid (EPA) and docosa-hexaenoic acid (DHA) increase both calcium absorption and accelerate calcium's delivery to the bones.

MYTH TWO:
BONES AND BRAINS ARE
NOT CONNECTED

Attention deficit disorder (ADD) and attention deficit hyperactivity disorder (ADHD) are the fastest-growing childhood learning problems in North America. ADD and ADHD refer to children, teens, and adults who are inattentive, impulsive, easily distracted, hyperac-tive, and unable to follow instructions. In November 2005, the *Journal of the American Academy of Child and Adolescent Psychiatry* published information that an astounding 5–8 percent of our children and teens, approximately 6 million in 2005, are believed to suffer from attention deficit.

Successful treatment of learning disabilities, ADD, and ADHD in childhood can help the next generation of teenagers from experiencing more serious problems— and save hundreds of thousands of adults from untold misery in the future.

The Bone–ADD, ADHD Connection

Most people have no idea that learning disabilities, ADD, and ADHD are closely connected to the quality of our bone health. Even though a few key minerals make up only 0.5 percent of the brain's weight, they are crucial ingredients that, like traffic signals, turn biological switches in the brain "on" and "off."

Calcium and magnesium are responsible for the quality of brain function and make up most of the mineral content of the brain. Calcium also interacts with potassium and sodium to balance nerve impulse activation and inactivation in the brain. Zinc is the third most important mineral in the brain. Zinc ignites electrochemical receptor and transmitter sites on the surface of neurons to encourage neurotransmission of thoughts, ideas, and impulses. Dr. Sidney V. Stohs, of Creighton University in Omaha, Nebraska, proved that zinc pushes the potentially harmful metals iron and copper out of brain communication neurons. Also vital, non-acidic forms of vitamin C (called calcium ascorbate) pull heavy metals like lead, mercury, cadmium, and aluminum out of the brain by wrapping them up in a process called chelation. Vitamin C is necessary to the brain's manufacture of dopamine, norepinephrine (adrenaline), and serotonin, three of the critical neurotransmitters involved in ADD and ADHD.

In ADD and ADHD the brain can become "water-logged" from excess fluids and communication or behavioral functions can become impaired and derailed. *Proanthocyanidins*, a member of a larger class of protective polyphenol compounds that we get from fruit and vegetables, especially in dark red and purple grapes, have a remarkable influence on learning disabilities, ADD and ADHD, and bone health.

Proanthocyanidins act as natural antihistamines to relieve the waterlogged brain. Dr. Jacques Masquelier found that they also inhibit the breakdown of the neurotransmitters dopamine, norepinephrine, and serotonin, which improves the communication and processing of information in the brain.

According to Lindsay Allen, Ph.D., a nutritional scientist from the University of California at Davis, children and teens do not have just one micronutrient deficiency, but many.

The world of ADD and ADHD therapy is bombarded by cure-of-the-week fads. But researchers are sorting out the best nutritional strategies to intervene and, according to a study in the February 2004 journal *Biochemicals*, positron emission tomography (PET) imaging measures energy production across the brain and shows that brain cell membranes that are highly enriched with calcium, magnesium, zinc, boron, vitamin C, fish oils rich in EPA and DHA essential fats, proanthocyanidins from grape seed and skins, and vitamin B6, B9, and B12 as found in a food-based, bone-building supplement, supply the cofactors that increase motivation, creativity, interest, attention span, and significantly reduce both hyperactivity and learning disabilities—naturally. Boost your bones, boost your brain!

MYTH THREE: "YOU SHOULD REST YOUR WEARY BONES"

Bones Are Not Static But a Clever Creation of Nature

Bone is a living organ that is constantly transforming as it repairs or replaces itself. The 206 bones that make up our skeleton are entirely renewed and replaced every seven to 10 years. The process of renewing and replacing bone is called remodeling.

Remodeling is vitally important for two reasons:

1. Daily bangs, bumps, bruises, and strains on bones cause tiny micro-fractures that need to be repaired with well-formed, healthy, new bone tissue.

2. Remodeling allows our bones to meet the various challenges or stresses that individuals place upon them such as the stronger bone development in the tennis player's racquet arm, the secretary's hands, the chef's fingers, the gardener's back, and the soccer player's feet and legs.

Bone Is a Pretty Amazing Living Tissue

We often think of bone as a sort of armor—the skull, for example, is a bony sphere that protects the delicate brain, and the ribs protect the heart, lungs, and organs from blows and injury. Yet, bone is the only organ that has microscopic cells, called *osteoblasts*, that are specifically designed to repair and rebuild. Bone also has microscopic cells called *osteoclasts*, whose sole purpose is to dissolve and break down bone at about 1,000th of an inch a day. At any given moment, you can have up to 8 million sites throughout your 206 bones, where small patches of old bone, or injured bone, are being dissolved and new bone being laid down. Each second, our bodies produce almost 2.5 million red blood cells inside the 9 oz of bone marrow our bones contain. Nutrients from our diet flow in and out of bone, dissolved in blood, to nourish bone growth and red blood cell development. If nutrients are in suboptimal supply, both our bones and red blood cells deteriorate quickly.

Osteocytes: Our Bones' Switchboard Operators

Our bones have an invisible, organized intelligence that, through communication feedback loops, tell the intestines to absorb or to stop absorbing calcium, the kidneys to excrete or to stop excreting calcium in the urine, and the parathyroid gland to take or to stop taking calcium from the bones.

Whenever bones are challenged or stressed, they grow stronger at the site of strain to withstand the functional, mechanical, weight-bearing load put on that location. "Bones have an adaptive response to a mechanical loading strain as from exercise or strenuous activity," states Susan E. Brown, Ph.D., in her book *Better Bones, Better Body*. The bone-maintenance crews are called basic multicellular units (BMUs) of which osteocytes are the communication organizers.

Make Bones Grow Strong and Healthy

Bones need the strain of exercise and a bone-building diet to perpetuate healthy bone-building and remodeling all life long for peak bone mass and perpetual bone repair.

Osteocytes, when their sense gauge registers stress or physiological strain, secrete an enzyme called glucose 6-phosphate dehydrogenase (G6PD), which in turn switches "on" RNA production or biosynthesis of anti-inflammatory prostaglandins 1 and 3, PGE1 and PGE3. Osteocytes continue this sequence of events by amplifying an extracellular protein called tenascin-C-transcription, which opens up calcium absorption channels and boosts the osteoregulatory (nutrient-absorption) response of osteoblast cells.

Using their body-wide communication network, osteocytes are strain- or weight-bearing sensors that evaluate the amount of new bone needed at any specific site. Buried within each bone membrane are 25,000 osteocytes per cubic millimeter—the size of a pinhead.

Osteocytes do an area-wide evaluation of where new bone needs to be formed through a vast communication network called the *"Bone-Building Internet."* Imagine the chaos if our 206 bones and their trillions of independent cells lacked the moment-to-moment communication coordination to build new bones—we would dissolve into a heap of jelly.

What Stops Us from Becoming One Solid Bone?

How intriguing bone-building is. For example, how do bones know when to stop renewing, replacing, and building? Feedback loops in the bone-building osteoblast cells, which control the intricate crystallization of bone, sense peak bone-repair and growth, and signal the osteocytes to turn "off" all biological switches for bone-building. Without these, we would be a heap of jelly or a solid, stone-like block!

MYTH FOUR:
ARE MEN REALLY THE STRONGER, MORE DOMINANT SEX?

It would seem by the latest research that history has not been quite accurate in its understanding of the sexes. Women have a decided advantage when it comes to living longer, healthier lives. Males are born with one X chromosome and one Y chromosome. Females are born with two X chromosomes.

Recent genetic research strongly indicates that the X chromosome is the stronger of the two when it comes to warding off disease and increasing longevity. Women worldwide outlive men, and in North America women live an average of 81.1 years compared with 75.1 years for men.

Dr. Barbara Migeon, a professor of genetics at the Institute of Genetic Medicine, Johns Hopkins University School of Medicine, wrote a special research article in 2006 called "X Advantage."

In the past, researchers concluded that male-female differences were limited to life experiences, hormones, or reproductive apparatus. Dr. Migeon states that, "What's been left out is the fundamental genetic differences between the sexes."

Dr. Migeon stresses that the difference originates in the fact that women come with two copies of the powerful X chromosome. "People think the X chromosome is only about sex, but it contains 1,100 genes that do all kinds of things from being involved in muscle function, bone function and blood clotting, to getting rid of cellular waste. It is a very active chromosome."

Female offspring receive an X chromosome from each parent, while male offspring receive an X chromosome from the mother and a comparatively "weak" Y chromosome from the father. The Y chromosome has a small amount of active DNA that is mainly responsible for the development of male characteristics. "So, if there is a mutation on the X chromosome, he is stuck with just this defective copy," Dr. Migeon points out. "However, females have two X chromosomes and if they have the same mutation, they have a back-up." At any one time, one of a woman's X chromosomes is switched "off," while the other remains active. But there is a downside to having the two X chromosomes and that is because the rare, simultaneous expression of both X chromosomes can leave women prone to autoimmune diseases such as lupus or scleroderma.

To the woman's great advantage, if she eats smart, exercises smart, supplements smart, and makes smart lifestyle choices, she can significantly reduce the risk of osteoporosis, type 2 diabetes, heart disease, and cancer in her lifetime. Her two X chromosomes give her a decided advantage.

Men need not feel defeated by this latest research. The Y chromosome gives men a powerful drive to succeed and accomplish any task they put their minds to. We as men must continue to be aware of our genetic tendencies and take the care and the time to feed our bodies healthfully, exercise dutifully, and limit the stressors in our lives that lead to major illness like heart disease, stroke, cancer, type 2 diabetes, and even the unsuspected, "silent epidemic" of osteoporosis. Eat smart, exercise smart, supplement smart, and make smart lifestyle choices!

MYTH FIVE:
MILK IS THE BEST SOURCE OF CALCIUM

It can come as a shock to learn that dairy products could actually contribute to bone loss and broken bones.

Dairy products may not be an ideal source of calcium, simply because the protein in milk may cause calcium to leach out of your bones. Ironically, epidemiological research has shown that populations throughout the world with the highest rate of osteoporosis (which includes Canada and the United States) also consume the highest amount of dairy foods. Populations that do not drink milk, but instead get their calcium from plant sources, have extremely low rates of osteoporosis.

Close to 40 percent of the world's population (15 percent of Caucasians) lack the enzyme lactase, meaning they are unable to digest lactose, the sugar in milk, and have adverse reactions to milk products.

In the United States (not in Canada) bovine growth hormone (rBGH) is injected into dairy cows to stimulate about 10 percent more milk than untreated cows. Monsanto, the manufacturer of rBGH (also known as BST), says about a third of the dairy cows in the United States have been injected with rBGH, although many dairy farmers resist. Unfortunately, milk from rBGH cows is mixed with cow's milk not injected with rBGH in large tanker trucks during transport, which means that a greater percentage of the milk supply has been tainted with the rBGH drug.

Furthermore, in both Canada and the United States dairy cows can be injected with antibiotics or steroids. A recent FDA survey, according to Professor Jane Plant, in her book *Your Life in Your Hands*, found antibiotics and other drugs in 51 percent of milk samples taken in 14 cities. Surprisingly, you are what you eat—ate!

Dr. Walter Willett, author of *Eat, Drink and Be Healthy: The Harvard Medical School Guide to Healthy Eating*, writing in *Science*, states, "Adult populations with low fracture rates generally consume few dairy products. Milk and other dairy products may not be directly equivalent to calcium from supplements."

The solution is to consume only fat-free yogurt, fat-free cottage cheese or skim milk labelled "organic" since these cows have not been treated with rBGH, antibiotics, or steroids and they are generally grass fed. Grass fed cows have 50 percent less saturated fat and their alkalinizing grass diet lowers the acidity of their stomachs, thus the meat and dairy we consume is more alkaline.

The Best Food Sources of Calcium

A study of the FDA's book *The Composition of Foods* makes it clear that the highest calcium content for whole foods are in foods from the oceans. Nova Scotia dulse, spirulina, chlorella, and kelp have the highest percentage of calcium listed in whole foods—from 0.86 percent calcium to 1.1 percent. The edible portions of most meat contain about 0.01 percent calcium and fluid whole milk 0.21 percent.

The *American Journal of Clinical Nutrition* published research by Dr. Heaney and Dr. Weaver (in edition 51) that showed calcium absorption from milk is approximately 32 percent, while calcium absorption from broccoli, kale, brussels sprouts, mustard greens, and turnip greens ranges from 40 percent to 64 percent.

BEYOND MYTHS:
THE BONE-BUILDING SOLUTION

Osteoporosis (OP) can strike all men, women, animals, and mammals with bony skeletons, including fish, whales, porpoise, birds, reptiles, and amphibians. It appears that OP has caused havoc in bone strength since the beginning of time. Whether it's a large shoulder bone, your vertebrae, a wrist, a finger, a knee or a little toe, each is a complex unit that makes strong stature, good posture, and fluid biomechanical movement possible.

My purpose in writing this book is to give safer, more effective alternatives for increasing many bone-building functions by informing the public and the medical community of the benefits of superior, daily nutrition; smart biomechanical exercise; and especially breakthrough supplementation solutions.

All you need is a new solution, a little commitment, and determination to keep your 206 bones and 143 joints healthy and strong, all life long.

A New Approach Emerges to Solve a Widespread Problem

The International Osteoporosis Foundation estimates that there are 75 million people in Europe, North America, and Japan with osteoporosis. Furthermore, 200 million more are developing osteoporosis now, but do not yet have any symptoms.

The time is ripe for a shift in the paradigm of OP prevention and treatment.

Instead of simply administering prescription drugs, many doctors are now actually halting and reversing the symptoms of OP. How? With eight safe, natural, inexpensive solutions you can use from the age of five to 90+, that can be neatly summed up as:

1. Daily using a comprehensive bone-building supplement beyond simple calcium to enhance healthy bone function, posture, balance, and movement to the maximum and give bone-repair some oomph!

2. Smartly following the ancient rules of color-coded eating to include colorful food components called polyphenols, which turn "on" biological switches for strong bone-building and turn "off" biological switches that supervise bone-breakdown.

3. Zeroing in on green vegetables rich in vitamin K1.

4. Daily consuming "friendly bacteria" like *Lactobacilli* and *Bifidobacteria* contained in a bone-building supplement, or from fat-free organic yogurt, or from

eating fermented foods like sauerkraut, miso, or apple cider vinegar to convert vitamin K1 to K2, which helps to successfully guide calcium into your 206 bones.

5. Using vitamin D3 from sunshine or a supplement to boost maximum nutrient absorption from the intestines and bone-building functions all life long.

6. Contrary to popular belief, we are not what we eat—but what we actually absorb! Daily include a phosphatide complex, which is a unique molecule that is both *hydrophilic* (attaches to water-soluble vitamins, minerals, and food compounds) and *lipophilic* (attaches to fat-soluble vitamins, minerals, and food compounds) from lecithin, which is derived from the soybean. It is the only food that enables both water-soluble and fat-soluble nutrients to be absorbed from the small intestine into the bloodstream at an accelerated rate.

7. Physically modifying, training, and rejuvenating your bones, balance, and fluid movement through daily core and strength-training exercises proven to improve your biomechanics and to cause bones to grow stronger at any age, all life long.

8. Eating an alkaline diet utilizing fresh, colorful salads, vegetables, and brightly colored fruit and berries. Fast foods and processed foods encourage an unhealthy "grab-and-feed" attitude and generally cause an acidifying effect in your body that is extremely corrosive to your 206 bones, 143 joints, 100 trillion cells, brain, arteries, heart, tooth enamel, and nails.

Learning to Use New Tools to Improve Bone Health

At the dawn of any new year, the world always carries the potential to be an appreciably healthier place. With new research and techniques being tried and new medical initiatives being launched, our tools and insights are better than ever. Now we must learn to put them to good use.

The Bill and Melinda Gates Foundation with the generous help of Warren Buffett took the lead in battling malaria, which kills 1 million people each year. In 2006, the foundation increased its already generous grants for research by $258 million, which means it provides more than a third of the world's entire malaria-research budget.

Things keep changing! As of 2006, U.S. food manufacturers must put the amount of insidious trans fatty acids, per serving size, on all food packaging. This is the result of many years of persistent, scientific research to prove that trans fats do accumulate in the lipid-soluble parts of the brain and heart cells, where they can become lethal. Institutions and businesses are learning from these insights, too. McDonald's, which has been publicly chastised for its role in creating the supersize culture in the first place, took supersizing off its menu in 2004 and 2005. McDonald's recently announced that it would begin putting nutritional information on the packaging of all its products in 2006. As an outside advisor, I recommended to McDonald's in the early 1990s that they add salads and veggie burgers to their menus. Furthermore, I highly suggested they use more tomatoes, onions, lettuce, and pickles on their burgers, and offer an option of a multigrain bun. My professional advice was rejected. No matter what, "in time all walls must fall." Even the American Heart Association in 2005 published guidelines for patients with coronary heart disease (CHD), recommending a consumption of fish and fish oil totaling 1 g a day of "mood-smart" EPA and "bone-smart" DHA. These EPA and DHA fatty acids also help to boost bone-building and increase your mood and memory power.

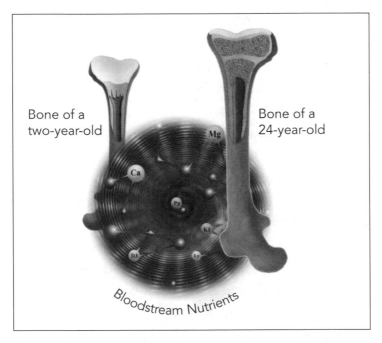

Figure 2.3: Bones Develop, Grow, and Change as We Age

From the moment of conception, our bones are developing, growing, and changing. The cartilage-like bone of a two-year-old must have sufficient bloodstream nutrients to grow into the strong bone of a 24-year-old.

No Bones About It—Ethical Calcium Researchers Abound

There has been an explosion in research on bone health. From osteopenia, osteoporosis, strong teeth and nails, calcium bioavailability and absorption, to the nutritional needs of healthy bones beyond just calcium, the optimistic, scientific breakthroughs of great researchers demonstrate the benefits of:

1. An alkalinizing, balanced nutritional strategy of three meals and two snacks a day based on brightly colored fresh produce

2. Quality lean protein daily to build the scaffolding for maximum bone mineral density (BMD), and bone strength and health

3. Reducing inflammation with EPA- and "bone-smart" DHA-rich fish oils that ramp up bone-building, enhance your good mood and brainpower

4. Encouraging vitamin D3 production from sunlight exposure on the skin or through supplementation as D3 accelerates calcium absorption into the body

5. Bone-building exercise and stress reduction build strong bones and give good balance

6. Vitamin K1 from green vegetables and yogurt cultures to convert K1 to active K2

7. Magnesium, phosphorus, and strontium boost bone-building

8. Folic-acid and vitamins B12 and B6 enhance bone repair

9. Bioavailable boron and silicon reinforce bone strength

10. "Molecular-targeted" bone-building supplements incorporate far more than calcium and vitamin D3

In this book you will be learning about the dramatic, new scientific research leading to unique and genuine bone-building breakthroughs.

Some Research Results Confirm What We Suspected—Some Are Counterintuitive

We live in an era that is bursting with information and many dizzying possibilities. Choices—both trivial and profound—confront us at every turn so that we can almost feel our brain cells and mental performances crackling and surging. From selecting the best mobile-phone plan to knowing which eggs to buy (Grain fed? White or brown? Free range? Omega-3 enriched?), surely there has never been a greater need to stay informed, alert, and healthy. How else could you remain focused, creative, and act with few or no glitches in your mental gymnastics and shrewd judgments?

Luckily for us, we also live in an age in which research is paying careful attention to both our mental and physical welfare. Research is showing us how to nurture and maintain our physical bodies and our mental faculties—from infancy through our "golden years"— and how to slow down what was once considered the inevitable declining spiral of our bone structure.

Some new findings are unexpected, even outright counterintuitive. Others confirm what our grandparents, parents, or we ourselves have always suspected:

- Grandpa was right—*"early to bed, early to rise."* Getting less than eight hours of sleep puts us in sleep debt, compromises our ability to concentrate effectively, and causes an acceleration in bone-breakdown.

- Our parents were right—*"laughter is the best medicine."* One hour of laughter opens our arteries by 22 percent and is equal to half an hour of hard cardiovascular exercise. Children laugh and giggle, on average, about 200 times a day, while adults average only 14 times a day.

- Grandma was right—*"fish really is brain food."* Fish can prevent depression and give us a big mood boost, plus it boosts healthy bone-building.

- A steaming cup of black coffee actually turbo-charges your mental acuity, creativity, and enthusiasm.

- Daily meditation physically transforms the brain's cerebral cortex and opens up our left prefrontal cortex, the site of peace, harmony, contentment, and fulfilled purpose—it counterbalances *frazzing*—ineffective multitasking, typically with the delusion that you are getting a lot done; the quality of the work, however, is poor.

- Some of the world's most creative and productive individuals simply refuse to subject their brains to "excess data streams." Meditation limits technological mental intrusions reducing inflammation in bone-forming and bone-repair cells.

- Physical exercise breaks down and removes gooey, sticky beta amyloid protein molecules from our brain and is equally important at boosting bone-repair.

- A long history of psychological research proved what one might expect: Performance declines as acute stress rises, causing bone-breakdown in relation to the increasing number of tasks juggled as you try to zip through your daily to-do list.

- Molecular biologists now understand the interactions between your diet and your DNA, and they are able to give you more personalized advice about what to eat and drink. For example, 10 to 20 percent of the population have a genetic variation that makes it harder for the body to absorb calcium in the presence of caffeine, thus increasing their risk of osteoporosis. Testing for this genetic variation costs about $250.00.

- Our mental performance, despite a few glitches with short-term memory, doesn't peak until midlife from 35–65, when the white matter in the loftiest part of the brain is thickest. Bones may also be able to stay strong for a lifetime.

- And most unexpected, but outright reassuring and comforting, recent research confirms that human bones, if nurtured properly, retain an astonishing degree of strength and growth capacity throughout life.

Beyond Calcium: Are Your Bones, Teeth, and Nails Getting Weaker or Stronger?

It's called the calcium paradox.

Dr. Walter Willet, chair of nutrition at the Harvard School of Public Health, states that, "countries with higher calcium intakes have the highest fracture rates, not the least." The simple question of logic seems coun-terintuitive. If your bones, teeth, and nails require calcium, then people who eat a lot of calcium-rich dairy products should have extra-strong bones, right? So why are hip fractures uncommon in Thailand, or broken ver-tebrae uncommon in Turkey, or wrist fracture rates low in southern California, while they soar in dairy-loving Europe, Canada, and most of the United States?

Remarkably, we have discovered three other crucial bone strengtheners that we are on even shorter supply than calcium: vitamin D3 to mobilize and ensure that calcium is absorbed into your body from the intestinal tract; bone-building exercise to stimulate bone-building cells into a "bone-strengthening spurt"; and vitamin K2 to chaperone calcium into bones and out of the arter-ies or kidneys, preventing hardening of the arteries and kidney stones.

The Calcium Paradox Unravelled

You know and understand that calcium must team up with a host of other essential nutrients, but how does this work? Research scientists have identified 40 vita-mins and minerals that your body needs for various tasks, from bolstering the brain and shoring up bones to keep them strong, to repairing cellular wear-and-tear. But as the calcium paradox suggests, they work much more subtly than drugs. Forgo your daily salad for a multivitamin pill and you will miss out on other com-pounds that fight cancer, protect the heart, boost your immune system, maintain bone integrity, and combat viral or bacterial infections.

"You can't just pop a vitamin C pill over a dark Belgium, double hot-fudge sundae and expect to cancel one and get great benefit from the other," says Dr. Alan Logan, author of the must-read *The Brain Diet*.

Please pay careful attention!

Instead of delivering predictable effects at exact particular doses, vitamins and minerals team up with other food constituents in complex ways we're just now beginning to understand. But never mistake the subtlety of these natural compounds and complexes for a lack of sheer power. Exciting new findings are pouring out of our research labs, linking long-neglected and unsuspected nutrients to everything from bone-building to cancer protection, diabetes, depression, and heart support.

What is most puzzling and increasingly clear is that in spite of our enormous and abundant food supply, we are still, by far and large, getting too little of many critical and crucial vitamins and minerals on a daily basis.

If you eat high-nutrient, natural, low-calorie foods daily, such as crisp salads, colorful vegetables, seasonal berries, melons, fresh fruit, essential fats, whole grains, nuts, seeds, legumes, herbs, spices, and lean protein from either animal or plant sources—and intelligently forgo the salty, sugary-sweet, calorie-intense fast foods, soft drinks, and junk foods, all enticingly and colorfully packaged—you help yourself to live well and quickly target some of our most common dietary deficiencies.

As the calcium paradox suggests, calcium on its own cannot shore up and bolster healthy bone-building every day of our lives—unless we are intentionally consuming many long-neglected compounds in whole, natural foods and biocompatible, "food-based" supplements to combine them into a bona fide bone-building team.

Beyond Calcium: Vitamin D3 Drives Bone Health

The *Tufts University Health and Nutrition Newsletter* in February 2006 ran an important headline, "Vitamin D Drives Bone Health." The article states that evidence of the important role that vitamin D3 plays in developing healthy bones continues to mount. "A recent Icelandic study has concluded, in fact, that if you are not getting enough vitamin D3, it may not matter how much calcium you consume," researchers stated. Jennifer Wider, M.D., from the Society for Women's Health Research, emphasizes that vitamin D works in the intestines to escort calcium into the bloodstream and also in the kidneys to help absorb calcium that would otherwise be excreted. Vitamin D3 enhances the ability of calcium to be absorbed into the osteoblast cells of bones. Most people do not know they are depleted in vitamin D3 because that has become their normal state. There are two blood tests your physician can use to measure your vitamin D3 levels—1,25(OH)D and 25(OH)D. Request the 25(OH)D, as it is a better marker of overall vitamin D3 status.

You require a minimum of 800–1,000 IU of vitamin D3 daily.

The New England Journal of Medicine reported a flawed study with skewed results in February 2006 that suggested taking calcium and 400 IU of vitamin D supplements did not enhance bone-building. The amounts of vitamin D used in this observational study were simply too low to absorb the calcium from the intestinal tract. Furthermore, if the calcium is not totally dissolved and absorbed because of a lack of dietary vitamin K2, probiotics, and insufficient vitamin D3, and not enough digestive acids in the stomach, the calcium could end up as kidney stones—not in our bones.

In the January 2006 issue of the journal *Carcinogenesis*, researchers at the University of Rochester Medical Center proved that vitamin D3 simultaneously reduced and decreased the activity of two enzymes, believed to play key roles in malignant tissue metastasis (the cathepsins and tissue inhibitor matrix metalloproteinase-1), that spread cancer cells. Dr. Lee and colleagues proved the anti-cancer benefits of 800 IU of vitamin D3 daily.

In the February 2006 edition of *The Journal of Clinical Investigation*, researchers showed that the biologically active form of vitamin D3 (1,25-dihydroxyvitamin D3) inhibited the production of a protein called c-Fos, which is important in the formation of osteoclast (bone-breakdown) cells. Therefore, when c-Fos is inhibited by vitamin D3, osteoclast development and activity is suppressed and the typical, accelerated bone loss after age 34 is slowed dramatically.

The Dynamic Duo: Vitamin D3 and Calcium

In May 2005, the *European Journal of Clinical Investigation* published some exciting and amazing research by two well-known Austrian researchers, Dr. Heidi Cross and Dr. Meinrad Peterlik, who demonstrated that higher levels of vitamin D3 and calcium must go together. Vitamin D3 can't do what it needs to do without adequate calcium, and vice versa.

Their research concluded: "Hypovitaminosis D (low vitamin D status) and low calcium intake is a widespread phenomenon in the adult population of Europe as well as North America . . . and an important public health problem because of numerous implications for increasing the development of osteoporosis, type 2 diabetes, rheumatoid arthritis, osteoarthritis, breast cancer, prostate cancer and colon cancer."

When they checked for calcium and vitamin D deficiencies in men and women, they were shocked to discover that 89 percent of adults are deficient in both calcium and vitamin D.

Their research highly encourages us to get at least 1,000 mg of absorbable, elemental calcium a day and 800–1,000 IU of vitamin D3, from food and supplements, to maintain bloodstream levels of vitamin D around 50 ng/mL, each and every day, all year round!

Early Lessons from Podravia and Istra

Podravia and Istra are rural districts of the former Yugoslavia. In the late 1960s and early 1970s, a remarkably ambitious study of their populations yielded valuable information about calcium and bone-building.

The people of Podravia traditionally raise dairy cows, and their calcium intake is high. These people spend a great deal of time inside barns. The people of Istra have the same genetic heritage, but that region grows more vegetables and grains, and calcium consumption typically is much lower. They spend more time outdoors in the sunshine, physically working hard.

Velimir Matkovic, M.D., and colleagues from the Medical School University of Zagreb in the former Yugoslavia wondered if these lifelong differences in eating habits and sun exposure would be reflected in the strength of their bone-building mass.

By checking diet histories from a sample of residents, the scientists learned that the average calcium intake of women in dairy-rich Podravia was 900 mg per day; in Istra, the average was only 400 mg per day. Meanwhile, for six years, they tracked the hospital records of 159,446 people from Podravia and 174,250 from Istra, checking for fractures.

The result: Women in Istra, whose normal diet was low in calcium, experienced 104 hip fractures during the six-year period. But women from the dairy-producing district of Podravia had 225 hip fractures. The results were published in the *American Journal of Clinical Nutrition* in 1979.

By reviewing this study today, when we know so much more about the importance of getting vitamin D3 and exercise along with calcium, we realize that the harder physical work and the extra vitamin D3 from sunshine, and the extra vitamin K1 from vegetables, helped the bone-building of the Istra women. They also ate fermented foods like sauerkraut and yogurt, which convert vitamin K1 to its biologically active form, K2. The people of Istra ate more color-coded vegetables, which are rich in polyphenols that support bone-building to the maximum because they make the body more alkaline, which, in turn, boosts and preserves bone-building quality.

Calcium and vitamin D are helpful to more than our bones. In June 2005, the *Archives of Internal Medicine* published research stating that 90 percent of all women experience premenstrual syndrome (PMS) at some point during their childbearing years. Calcium and vitamin D3 reduce PMS by almost 40 percent. Osteoporosis declines by 60 percent and some cancers by 50 percent with the adequate amounts of calcium and vitamin D3 added to the diet. Younger women take note.

> Calcium, by the way, does a lot more than just build strong bones.

Calcium is also critical for transmitting nerve impulses and maintaining a regular heartbeat. It stimulates crucial hormone secretions and activates enzymes. Combined with vitamin D3, it may even help to protect against colon, breast, and prostate cancers—reducing risk by an astonishing 50 percent.

Molecular-Targeted Bone-Building Supplements

An ancient biological dance happens to minerals, trace minerals, vitamins, protein, and phytonutrients (disease-reducing compounds in all vegetation) once they enter the cells of your body. In nature, the molecules of minerals are arranged in random clusters. Once these mineral and trace mineral molecules find their way into your 100 trillion cells, however, they become highly organized. Minerals and trace minerals exist within the microenvironment of bone-building cells in a complex, multilayered, organized structure.

Imagine that the minerals and trace minerals in food or a bone-building supplement are like a container of alphabetical letters all mixed up. After you consume them, if you look inside the living cells in your bones with a high-resonance microscope, you would see an activated bone-building construction of words, sentences, and paragraphs called "molecular-targeting," busy zeroing in on the creative bone-building process.

A NOBEL PRIZE FOR BREAK-THROUGH MINERAL RESEARCH

Minerals function as cofactors for literally thousands of different metabolic enzymes. Magnesium drives energy-production reactions and assists heart muscle tissue in creating contraction and expansion rhythms. Macronutrient minerals like calcium, magnesium, and phosphorus combine with a broad spectrum of micronutrient trace minerals like zinc, copper, boron, manganese, and silicon to form bone-building, skeletal structures.

Minerals should always be taken together because they compete for absorption sites in the small intestine and unsuccessful competition may cause a depletion of some minerals. Calcium, as an example, should always be taken in a 1.5 to 1 ratio with magnesium in order to guard against magnesium depletion and to improve calcium absorption and utilization. Minerals like calcium and magnesium must be escorted successfully across the intestinal barrier and into the bloodstream for transport to each living bone cell.

Günter Blobel, M.D., from Rockefeller University, won the Nobel Prize in medicine in 1999 when he discovered that small protein peptide chaperones (guides) not only guide protein into tissue, but chaperone and guide proteins to where they are needed. Because of this breakthrough, a whole new world of biophysics and biochemistry has started to unfold. Dr. G. Alfred Gilman and Dr. Martin Rodbell won a Nobel Prize in medicine for specifically describing the role that protein folding plays in intracellular, cell-to-cell communication or cell signal transduction pathways.

Other research scientists have shown that this same protein chaperone system guides minerals to the correct receptor sites, deeply embedded in the membrane of each cell, especially bone cells. Plants, animals, and humans use this same common system of protein chaperones to deliver minerals, over secure pathways, to cells. Consequently, calcium, magnesium, zinc, copper, boron, selenium, iron, and silicon that are bound to proper chaperones appear to be the most highly bioavailable in humans and contribute to maximize bone-building.

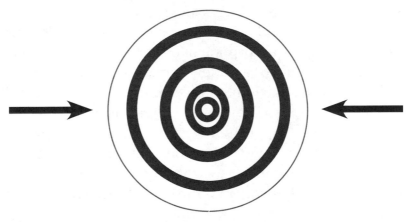

Figure 2.4: Molecular-Targeting

The Institute of Medicine, the National Academy of Sciences, the USDA, and Health Canada have established panels of experts to review micronutrient daily requirements. The expert panels have recently begun establishing higher upper limits and optimal levels for micronutrients needed for bone-building and maintaining good health. It has only recently been established within the scientific research community that diet alone may not supply all the micronutrients we need daily. Correcting micronutrient deficiencies requires optimum doses, higher than previously recommended, to ignite a sluggish metabolic system. Bruce Ames, Ph.D., Department of Molecular and Cell Biology, University of California at Berkeley, states that "Metabolic harmony requires an optimum intake of each micronutrient: deficiency distorts metabolism in numerous and complicated ways, many of which may lead to cellular damage."

Even the tiniest deficiencies could cause subtle and undetected disruption in peak cellular and bone-building well-being. Roy Walford, M.D., a world-renowned researcher who was at the University of California, Los Angeles Medical School, stated that "Simple, biological activity involves the coordinated activity of billions of cells, countless biochemical pathways and many small protein peptides, and their associated cell-to-cell communications. It may well be that relatively small daily dietary deficiencies that are dismissed as causing only minor changes to the activity of a single cell will, along with many other similar minor effects, have a measurable and potentially damaging cumulative influence on cellular functioning and energy production." This is how optimum bone-building functions decrease and derail, silently beginning at about age 24 and starting to show physical signs by age 34.

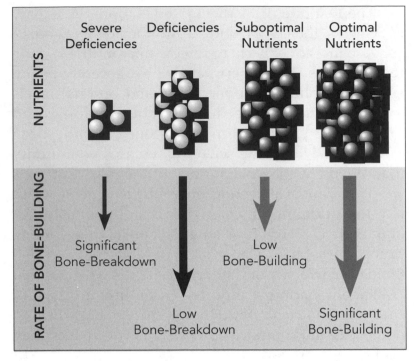

Figure 2.5: The Effect of Various Degrees of Nutrient Deficiencies on Bone-Building

Creating a Stronger Structure with Ancient Wisdom

New, scientific breakthrough lab results routinely demonstrate that specialized multiple forms of calcium, piggybacked with 19 other critical and key micronutrients, are absorbed significantly better—by 200–1,500 percent better—than the more commonly used and questionable calcium supplements. These suboptimal forms of calcium include calcium carbonate, calcium citrate, calcium lactate, calcium gluconate, calcium diphosphate, microcrystalline hydroxyapatite complex (MCHC) (ground cow bones), dolomite, and bonemeal.

The most effective forms of calcium have a specific frequency of quantum energy that is highly recognized by absorption sites throughout the small intestine. They are taken up by the bloodstream quickly because they do not require stomach acids to be absorbed.

Zero in on Bone-Building with Targeted Supplements

Calcium bisglycinate, calcium formate, and calcium citrate-malate have been shown to interact with one another incredibly effectively. They exchange energy at electro-absorption sites and drive absorption gradients sensitive to voltage, which enhances cell-to-cell pathways and boosts intracellular communication.

These three multifunctional sources of calcium, piggybacking with many other key micronutrients also orchestrate specific bone-building tissue responses in an ever-changing cellular environment—at all ages.

These three companion calciums and their micronutrient cofactors when combined are called "molecular-targeted" supplements because their transfer from the intestines to bones is smooth and harmonious. Broad-spectrum supplementation boosts bone-building because the individual elements piggyback upon each other in perfect synergism. These calciums and micronutrients play a vital role in our bones' gene expression and in the bidirectional communication between living *osteoblast* (bone-building) and *osteoclast* (bone-breakdown) cells in bones. This means that target supplementation is particularly effective in stabilizing bone-repair systems and in initiating bone-building.

This new, effective osteoporosis-fighting supplement can halt, reverse, and possibly even cure degenerative osteoporosis. Based on the most recent and cutting-edge medical research, these forms of calcium cause bone-building osteoblast cells to communicate at optimum levels even in subacute chronic osteoporosis.

Bone-building micronutrients ultimately increase the communication between osteoblast and osteoclast cells, giving a dynamic vitality or life force to bone, teeth, skeletal structure, posture, and fluid biomechanical movements, in an amazingly short time.

When purchasing any bone-building supplement from your local natural food store, insist on a formula that contains the types and amounts of macronutrients, micronutrients, minerals, vitamins, and phytonutrients listed in Chapter 5.

Meanwhile, research continues to reveal the powerful ability of exact food components to build or rebuild your bones, teeth, nails, posture, and movement while modifying other potential disease processes such as reducing plaque buildup in arteries and reducing heart attack risks.

THE RENEWAL ISSUE FOR BONES

This book offers incredible new strategies for moving beyond the ineffective and imbalanced forms of minerals developed in the 1990s—and still used today—that cause chemical disturbances and an improper series of molecular exchanges, as well as failing to properly renew, regulate, or maintain superior bone health. They also may cause kidney stones.

The ultimate bone-building strategy works in conjunction with the ancient power and wisdom of your body's innate ability to heal, restore, and regenerate.

BONE MINERAL DENSITY

Bone Mineral Density (BMD) mysteriously begins to disappear in almost everyone from age 34 onward. The eventual large-scale loss of bone can be intimidating. Look at your grandmother and grandfather or mother and father. If you want to improve the way you will look, feel, and move at their age, you must alter your lifestyle now! You can prevent this decline in bone strength and bone volume, which is accepted by the majority of the population to be a natural part of the aging process. It is not! Follow the step-by-step, medically proven dietary, moderate exercise, and supplemental guidelines in this book and you can tangibly enhance bone-building and reverse bone deterioration right away for better structure, posture, and healthy appearance. Stand tall, all life long.

> Now that you understand that your bone cells communicate in a harmonious rhythm, you can help orchestrate that rhythm by sending them life-supporting micronutrient messages to improve the bidirectional "cross-talking" between osteoblast (bone-builder) cells and osteoclast (bone-breakdown) cells.

"It is confidence in our bodies, minds and spirits that allows us to keep looking for new adventures, new directions to grow in, and new lessons to learn—which is what life is all about."

—Oprah Winfrey

Are You or Your Children at Risk of Osteoporosis?

Take the One-Minute Osteoporosis Risk Test

1. I'm over 50 years of age.
   ❏ Yes   ❏ No

2. My health is "poor" or "fair."
   ❏ Yes   ❏ No

3. Have either of your parents broken a hip after a minor fall or bump?
   ❏ Yes   ❏ No

4. Have you broken a bone after a minor fall or bump?
   ❏ Yes   ❏ No

5. Have you lost more than 1 inch in height?
   ❏ Yes   ❏ No

6. Do you smoke cigarettes, a pipe, cigars, or marijuana at least three times a week?
   ❏ Yes   ❏ No

7. Do you have more than one drink of alcohol several times a week?
   ❏ Yes   ❏ No

8. Do you exercise five days a week, doing both aerobic and anaerobic exercises?
   ❏ Yes   ❏ No

9. Do you average 15 minutes daily of unprotected sunshine on your skin or daily take 800 IU of supplemental vitamin D3?
   ❏ Yes   ❏ No

10. Women, did you start menopause before 45?
    ❏ Yes   ❏ No

11. Men, did you start andropause before 55?
    ❏ Yes   ❏ No

12. Do you experience diarrhea, digestive problems, or candida?

    ❑ Yes   ❑ No

13. Daily, do you eat 6 cups of fresh salad and vegetables, plus two or three pieces of fruit?

    ❑ Yes   ❑ No

14. Daily, do you eat 1 cup of unsweetened yogurt or 2 cups of milk?

    ❑ Yes   ❑ No

15. Do you use a bone-building supplement (not just calcium) five days a week?

    ❑ Yes   ❑ No

16. Do you avoid pop, colas, sweetened fruit juice, or artificial fruit-flavored drinks?

    ❑ Yes   ❑ No

17. Daily, do you eat green vegetables or salads or "green drinks" for vitamin K?

    ❑ Yes   ❑ No

18. Have you taken corticosteroids (cortisone, prednisone, steroids) or antibiotics or thyroid or cancer medication for more than three months?

    ❑ Yes   ❑ No

Scoring Key:

"Red flag," very high alert:	More than 6 Yes answers and 10 No
"Orange flag," medium alert:	More than 7 Yes answers and 9 No
"Green flag," very low alert:	More than 8 Yes answers and 8 No
"Red flag" for children:	More than 2 Yes answers and 10 No

It seems incredible that each of us can reach for and achieve a more fulfilled, content, serene, and happier life with optimum performance levels in our mental, physical, emotional, and spiritual domains. I want you to attain this!

> Your life is not a spectator sport—dare to make it better with improved stature, posture, and movement.

Can you be creatively adaptable to your daily food, supplement, and lifestyle choices? If you can, your immune system, brainpower, structural bone strength, posture, fluid biomechanical movements, elevated mood, and spiritual awareness will thank you by keeping you healthy, and your 100 trillion cells will dance with authentic joy. They will talk to you with a constant buzz of available energy, ready to respond to your daily needs.

I encourage you to put these incredible research breakthroughs into your personal toolbox and learn to quickly put them to good use, because our amazing tools are now better than ever.

CHAPTER **3**

The Living Micro-Architecture of Bone

THE MICRO-ARCHITECTURE OF BONE

Our bodies contain over 206 bones. Press your finger on your forehead, your forearm, or hip, and you can explore your bones through your skin. The word "skeleton" comes from the Greek *skeletos*, which means "hard and dried up." But bone is alive, and, like all living tissue, it daily and continuously renews itself. Bone-building requires good nutrition and proper exercise to stay in good health.

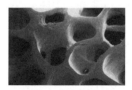

Natural healthy bone with strong honeycombs

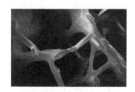

Osteoporotic bone that is thinner, weaker, and more prone to fracture

Figure 3.1: Microscopic Photos of Bone

Source: Reproduced with permission from Journal of Bone Mineral Research 1 (1986): 15–21 by the American Society for Bone Mineral Research.

BONE: A LIVING TISSUE

Are you at risk for osteoporosis? We are all vulnerable to osteoporosis, and become more so as we get older. The 2004 Surgeon General's Report states that by 2020, 50 percent of all North Americans over 50 years of age will have weak bones and osteoporosis unless they make changes to their diet and lifestyle now!

Bone is a remarkable tissue with the same strength as cast iron, while remaining as light as wood. It can adapt to its functional demands and repair itself. Bone is living tissue made up of two major types, *trabecular bone* (the spongy honeycomb interior) and *cortical bone* (the solid, smooth outside coating).

The skeleton can rejuvenate and rebuild itself throughout life. When old, worn-out, or damaged bone is removed, the microscopic osteoblast (bone-building) cells come in and replace it. If you do not have adequate bone-building micronutrients and exercise daily, then when the new bone is deposited in the remodeling process, the amount of bone deposited by the osteoblast cells is just a little less than the amount of bone removed by the microscopic osteoclast (bone-breakdown) cells.

This means that there will be a little less bone each time this internal renovation takes place. Over many years, the dynamic bone-building equilibrium derails and skeletal mass and structure become less and less.

Over the last decade, as dramatic new scientific research techniques have become more sophisticated, our ability to learn about the complexities of bone-building has accelerated. Now scientists are discovering that the healthy growth of our 206 bones and 143 joints is far more complicated and ongoing than previously supposed. For example, bone loss has now been shown to have clear implications for dental health. As well, osteoporosis can begin in younger people, and men, too, must be vigilant in protecting their bone health, as will become clear in the following sections.

WEAK BONES, WEAK TEETH

"The evidence is becoming clearer and clearer—osteoporosis can impact your smile due to increased tooth loss and periodontal disease," according to Dr. Michael Bolognese, DDS, chairman of the Mid-Atlantic Osteoporosis Board.

Recent studies are beginning to detail the relationship between bones and teeth. For example, one report states that in cases of severe periodontal disease, individuals with osteoporosis suffer more tooth loss than similar non-osteoporotic patients. Another study states that people with high bone mineral density retain their teeth longer than people with low bone mineral density despite having deep gum pockets around the teeth.

Increased tooth loss is related to bone loss. The first research to prove this was published back in December 1996 in the journal *Calcified Tissue International*. Researchers concluded that:

> *Increased systemic bone loss may be a risk factor for tooth loss by contributing to the resorption of tooth-supporting alveolar bone (jaw bones that anchor your teeth). For each 1 percent per year lost in bone mineral density (BMD), relative risks of losing a tooth were significantly elevated. These results provide support for a role in systemic bone loss in the development of tooth loss!*

WEAK BONES, BRITTLE NAILS, POOR TEETH, AND YOUR DIGESTION

Strong digestion and good assimilation are essential for proper nutrient utilization, and in no case is this more true than with mineral metabolism. When we speak of calcium intake and calcium requirements, for example, we must remember that only a portion of the calcium we ingest is absorbed; the rest is excreted in the stool, urine, and sweat. Adults absorb anywhere between 15–30 percent of the calcium they ingest, depending on age, need, digestion, endocrine health, and other factors.

Anything that limits the absorption of calcium or any other mineral is detrimental to bone. Anything that increases mineral absorption benefits bone, and calcium is not the only mineral of importance. Proper vitamin absorption is also essential. For example, poor B12 absorption appears to play a role in bone health. Mayo Clinic researchers report that those with anemia have reduced bone mineral density and increased bone fracture incidence in comparison with the general community. Patients with pernicious anemia were found to have a double incidence of hip and spinal fractures and nearly a threefold increase in wrist fractures. Numerous studies now point to the bone-building value of strong digestion and good absorption.

Various osteoporosis researchers, in fact, now propose that malabsorption of calcium, magnesium, zinc, boron, silicon, etc., is often a major cause of thin, weak bones. One very important digestive weakness that hinders calcium absorption is low stomach hydrochloric acid (HCL). Without adequate stomach acid, our food is poorly digested and absorption of many nutrients, including calcium, iron, folic acid, and vitamins B6 and B12 is limited. Calcium, for example, must be in a soluble ionized form for absorption. This requires an acidic environment within the stomach, provided by adequate HCL.

Dr. Jonathan Wright, a well-known author and practicing physician, reports that the majority of his patients with osteoporosis suffer from insufficient HCL. Other research supports this finding. As early as 1941, people suffering jawbone loss were found to have one-half the HCL level of those without jawbone loss. In another study from 2005, investigators reported that 40 percent of postmenopausal women had no basal gastric acid secretion. Since exhaustion of HCL-producing cells within the stomach occurs with prolonged stress, it is likely that more HCL deficiency exists today than ever before.

A common hydrochloric acid deficiency might help explain the conflicting data around calcium supplementation and osteoporosis prevention. The confusion and controversy might well center on the issue of poor calcium absorption due to low hydrochloric acid. Most studies which show no beneficial effect of added calcium, used calcium supplements in the form of calcium carbonate. Calcium carbonate is poorly digested without adequate hydrochloric acid and thus of little use to those with weak digestion. When the more absorbable forms of calcium—such as calcium bisglycinate, formate, or citrate-malate—are administered, beneficial results are reported since they do not require stomach acids for them to be dissolved and absorbed.

If you have flatulency, gas, bloating, and indigestion, use three plant-sourced digestive enzyme capsules with each meal. You can also drink 1 tbsp of organic apple cider vinegar stirred in 4 oz of water 15 minutes before each meal to raise your stomach's hydrochloric acid levels. Another tip is to squeeze a little fresh lemon or lime juice on your foods or in your drinking water, especially before a meal.

OSTEOPOROSIS IS SHOWING UP AT YOUNGER AGES

Cross-cultural studies show that throughout the world most individuals lose bone mass as they age. The remaining bone, however, is healthy and capable of constant self-repair. This is normal aging bone loss, but this process leaves one with bones sufficiently dense and strong to withstand the stress and strain of daily activity. In osteoporosis, however, bone loss goes beyond that of normal aging and becomes accelerated.

More and more we are finding that even the young are not free from the specter of osteoporosis. Currently the disease is widely documented among young people. Among the groups most affected are anorexic individuals, training ballet dancers and other athletes who under-consume nutrients in an effort to remain very slim, and young people addicted to computer games who get no exercise or sunshine on their skin. Women who suffer from menstrual irregularities, those who have under-gone ovary and/or uterus removal, and persons on long-term steroid therapy are also affected. Dr. Lazarro, a radiologist at Upstate Medical Center in Syracuse, New York, is one of the many clinical practitioners to notice this recent trend. He reports they are finding a growing number of young women and young men with excessively low bone mass.

MALE CALL

Today there is a lack of awareness in young men about the "silent epidemic" of osteoporosis, and many still remain uninformed regarding the serious implications of their potential for fragility fractures of the wrist, vertebrae, and hip. Despite our revolutionary new view and insights to optimal health, the hallowed consensus among men is that they shouldn't worry about weak bones.

Figure 3.2 shows that the hip fracture rate for men worldwide, measured in the millions, will silently increase 200 percent by 2020. The implications for men are mind-boggling. Unfortunately, most men do not realize that the "silent epidemic" of osteoporosis affects them, or that their bones are becoming thinner, more porous, and brittle during their adult life. Yet, men in their twenties, thirties, forties, fifties, and sixties now have the potential to stop this "silent epidemic."

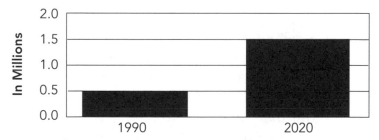

Figure 3.2: Hip Fracture Rate for Men Worldwide

Studies suggest that men are less likely than women to implement preventive health strategies, like a bone-building supplement, before they get sick. It makes much more sense to start while bone density is normal.

Men Are Less Diagnosed for Osteoporosis, But Their Rates Are Growing

A difference in men and women's bone remodeling probably explains why fractures occur less commonly in men. While bone is being remodeled in the honeycomb interior (trabecular marrow), new cells are being deposited, like a coat of paint, on the outside surface of the bone. The amount of new cortical bone deposited on the outside surface is about three times more in men than in women. This increases bone size, and so maintains the strength of the wider bone, as well as offsetting internal bone loss.

Why men are able to deposit more bone than do women is not known. It may be because they have more of the hormone testosterone, but this has not been proven. Yet, osteoporosis is a serious health problem in men. Part of the problem may be that when a man enters the doctor's office, the doctor thinks about checking for cardiovascular disease, lipids, stress, hypertension, alcohol or tobacco abuse, and prostate, lung, or bowel cancer, but rarely or never about osteoporosis and fractures. In fact, fewer than 5 percent of men with osteoporosis and fractures are investigated or treated even though a prevalent fracture is a clear predictor of future fractures.

One in four men over 50 will have a bone fracture that will reduce the quality of their lives, their mobility, their independence, and their life span, according to the International Osteoporosis Foundation. Health care providers should routinely check men over 50 for early signs of osteoporosis such as stooped posture, stiff joints, sore bones, and eroding tooth enamel.

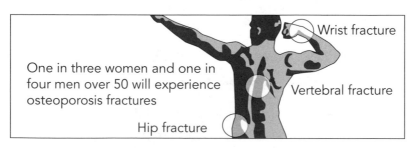

Figure 3.3: Common Sites of Fracture

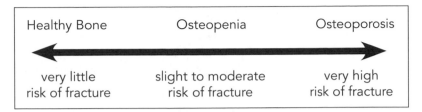

Figure 3.4: Osteopenia Can Improve or Decline

BONE FRACTURES

By far, the fracture that causes the most misery, pain, and disability in osteoporosis is the hip fracture, which occurs at the top of the thighbone or femur. It almost always occurs in a fall, usually from no higher than a standing height.

Hip fractures increase dramatically in women after the age of 65 and in men after the age of 70, with progressive increases in risk with advancing age. Because hip fractures require surgical repair, there is also the threat of surgical complications. The risk of dying in the year following a fracture is 20 percent higher. Of course, hip fractures are by no means the only concern. Pelvic fractures can also occur in a fall. Wrist fractures are common, but, fortunately, they respond well to casting, although they sometimes require surgical repair.

> The medical expense for treating broken bones from osteoporosis is as high as $19 billion U.S. each year in North America alone.

Rib fractures are also common. When osteoporosis exists, ribs can fracture as a result of the simplest of actions—coughing, sneezing, banging into something, or even from a tight hug.

VERTEBRAL FRACTURES

Vertebral fractures occur in the bones in the vertebral column. This is a piece of cube-shaped bone that projects forward toward the stomach from the spinal cord that you can feel when you run your hand along your back. These fractures do not usually require any casting, splinting, or surgical intervention and heal on their own.

But often chronic back pain sets in as the vertebrae compress down on each other. The person becomes very hunched over, losing height and developing the so-called dowager's hump deformity.

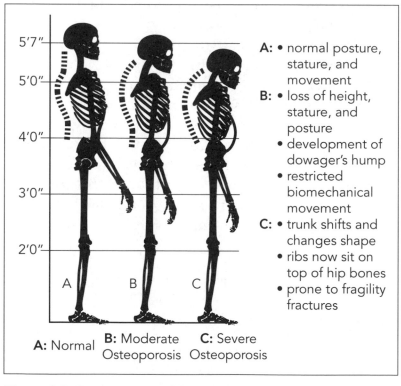

A: • normal posture, stature, and movement

B: • loss of height, stature, and posture
• development of dowager's hump
• restricted biomechanical movement

C: • trunk shifts and changes shape
• ribs now sit on top of hip bones
• prone to fragility fractures

A: Normal   B: Moderate Osteoporosis   C: Severe Osteoporosis

Figure 3.5: Consequences of Osteoporosis

OUR BLOODSTREAM MAINTAINS EXACT CALCIUM CONCENTRATIONS

The average female body has about 1,000 gm or 2.2 lbs of calcium and the average male about 1,200 gm or 2.6 lbs. Nearly 99 percent of the calcium is in our bones, teeth, and nails, and less than 1 percent is in body fluids. Of that 1 percent, about half is ionized and physiologically active, and the other half non-ionized and physiologically inert, mostly bound to the protein albumin.

Some of the calcium in the bones is in a form that is rapidly exchangeable and is available when needed to maintain proper levels of calcium in the bloodstream. Calcitonin, osteocalcin, and matrix G1a protein (MGP), along with parathyroid hormone, are the main regulators of "on" and "off" switches that control the flow of calcium into and out of our 206 bones. These regulators are ignited by vitamin K2 and they maintain bloodstream calcium at a normal concentration of 10 mg per 100 mL of blood. The inflow and outflow of calcium from bones is called the biomineralization process.

CAN YOUR BONES BE TESTED?

For some people the first sign of osteoporosis is when they break a bone easily or when they realize that they are getting shorter. Don't wait until that happens to find out if you have osteoporosis. You can have a *bone density test* to determine how solid your bones are. Your doctor may suggest a type of bone density test called a DEXA-scan (dual-energy X-ray absorptiometry) if you are 50 or older or if he or she thinks you are at risk for osteoporosis.

The DEXA-scan will determine your risk for a fracture or a broken bone: It could show that you have normal bone density, or it could show that you have low bone mass or even osteoporosis.

Should You Be Concerned about Radiation Exposure When You Have a Bone Density Test?

Excessive radiation exposure can cause cancer and other serious medical problems. Fortunately, bone density can be tested with only minimal radiation—so little that the technician can safely remain in the room.

All of us are exposed to radiation from environmental sources (including the sun and the ground we live on); most adults also have some exposure from medical procedures. Radiation exposure is usually measured in millirems (or mrems). Here are a few examples:

Radiation Source	Approximate Exposure (in mrems)
Environment (in North America)	0.5–1.5 per day
SXA (single X-ray absorptiometry)	1–2
DEXA (dual/energy X-ray absorptiometry)	1–3
RA (radiographic absorptiometry)	5
Coast-to-coast flight	5
Standard chest X-ray	25
Full dental X-ray	200–300
Computer tomography (CT) scan	10,000

Body scans are one of the latest health fads. A blizzard of media attention has healthy people flocking to "scan centers" to get their bodies scanned. The concept is terrific. State-of-the-art machines known as CTs (computed tomography) "slice" internal organs into wafer-thin serial images, which are then viewed on a computer screen. CT scans quickly reveal cancer, heart disease, osteoporosis, and more. It is great except for one thing—radiation—and lots of it. A whole body scan is equivalent to almost 1,000 X-rays. Radiation damage to DNA is never completely repaired. Never get a full body or chest CT scan unless you have serious risk factors.

COMMON DRUGS USED TO TREAT OSTEOPOROSIS

- *Evista (also known as Raloxifene) (SERM/Selective Estrogen Receptor Modulators)*

  Potential side effects experienced with SERMs are hot flashes, leg cramps, fever, or flu-like symptoms and/or increased incidence of infections, headaches, joint pain, indigestion, abdominal pain, insomnia, urinary/gynecological problems, dizziness, sinusitis, and weight gain.

- *Calcimar, Miacalcin (subcutaneous injectable calcitonin, and nasal spray calcitonin)*

  Potential side effects experienced with calcitonin spray are nasal irritations, runny nose, nosebleeds, itching, hives, difficulty breathing, swelling of lips, tongue, or face. With injectable calcitonin, they are nausea, vomiting, skin rash and/or flushing, and allergic reactions.

- *Forteo (injectable parathyroid hormone)*

  Potential side effects experienced with Teriparatide (Forteo) are joint pain, headaches, leg cramps, hypertension, angina, shortness of breath, nausea, various digestive problems, dizziness, depression, insomnia, fatigue, rhinitis, skin rash, and sweating.

- *Fosamax, Actonel, Boniva (oral bisphosphonates)*
  Aredia, Zometa (injectable bisphosphonates)

  Potential side effects experienced with bisphosphonates include heartburn and various digestive problems, allergic reactions, esophageal ulcer, headaches, joint/muscle pain or cramps, and osteonecrosis (death of the jawbone). This is a condition in which the bone tissue in the jaw fails to heal after minor trauma such as a tooth extraction, causing the bone to be exposed.

Drug-Induced Nutrient Deficiencies: Drugs Are Helpful, But ...

In 2005 Dr. Frederic Vagnini, M.D., and Dr. Barry Fox, Ph.D., published a well-researched book, *The Side Effects Bible: The Dietary Solution to Unwanted Side Effects of Common Medications*. Their book's emphasis is that pharmaceutical drugs perform many miracles every day, from controlling diabetes to containing virulent infections like the H5N1 bird flu.

However, it is important to remember that all drugs—even the simple and ubiquitous aspirin—have side effects. Perhaps 30 percent of pharmaceutical side effects are the direct result of drug-induced nutrient deficiencies. In other words, a drug *"robs"* you of one or more nutrients, or other helpful phytonutrients, and this sudden loss of super-critical nutrients causes side effects. Often, using a high-quality supplement can ameliorate or eliminate the side effects by restoring or compensating for the nutrient loss caused by a drug.

Most research scientists agree that the only solution to averting drug-induced nutritional deficiencies is to replace the depleted nutrients daily through:

1. using a "molecular-targeted," comprehensive bone-building supplement

2. deliberately and conscientiously consuming a large variety of brightly color-coded, "cell-friendly" fruits, vegetables, herbs, spices, and unprocessed whole grains

3. avoiding processed fast foods full of salt, fat, sugar, artificial sweeteners, excess calories, artificial colors, and taste enhancers that also promote a very unhealthy "grab-and-feed" mentality

4. avoiding smoking

5. avoiding or using alcohol in moderation.

ARE YOU IMPROVING YOUR BONE-BUILDING FUNCTIONS EVERY DAY?

One dogma about bone health has remained sacred until recently. The belief was that an osteoporotic bone cell once lost was gone forever. Thus older bones could not regenerate themselves. Experts believed any bone-density weakness was irreparable. Now, thanks to a group of visionary medical researchers, that idea has bit the dust, leading to thrilling new prospects of bone regrowth, recovery, and rejuvenation.

- You renew almost 1.75 million bone cells a second, 100 million cells a minute, and 150 billion bone-building cells a day, all of which dictate your bone mineral density (BMD).

- A study published in *The New England Journal of Medicine* was the first to prove that acute stress—as well as past or current depression—lowers BMD by 6 percent at the spine and up to 14 percent at the hip. A Mayo Clinic study found a significant positive correlation between BMD and muscle strength in those individuals who do weight-resistance and core muscle exercises.

- Early prevention or inhibition of age-related bone loss in men and women has never been easier! Nutritional interventions and exercise are nontoxic and far less expensive than any other treatment option. And they work! For example, in a study of 72 osteoporotic people comparing the use of vitamin K2 to a first-generation bisphosphonate drug, no difference was found in the bone fracture rate after 24 months.

GET A HEAD START ON IMPROVING YOUR BONE HEALTH

Unquestionably, scientists find a startling difference in bone cells of animals and people who are fed calcium-rich diets, vitamin D3, vitamin K1, magnesium, boron, silicon, isoflavones, and the micronutrient trace minerals copper, zinc, and manganese, and who also exercise regularly. They have healthy bones that are 40–60 percent stronger, denser, and more flexible than improperly nourished bones, which are all too often simply taken for granted. Truly we have entered a new miracle age with our bones, teeth, and nails bursting with the promise of unprecedented strength and lifelong health. All of us alive today can become the beneficiaries of this new knowledge!

Intriguingly, researchers have found that supplementation with the hormones DHEA and melatonin appear to enhance new bone formation, boost bone-repair systems, and inhibit excessive bone-breakdown.

Dehydropiandrosterone (DHEA)

DHEA is produced in the adrenal cortex. It is then rapidly converted into its sulfated form, DHEA-S, which is the primary form circulating in the bloodstream. Peak levels occur during the mid-twenties; after that, levels decrease rapidly and yearly until they are almost nonexistent by the time men and women reach their mid-eighties. DHEA begins to decline more quickly after age 34.

The lack of DHEA-S has been closely associated with weak bones, osteoporosis, loss of libido, and aging. A growing body of scientific research suggests that another important function of DHEA is to reduce and balance elevated levels of the stress hormone cortisol. Lowering cortisol levels gives a big boost to bone-repair and bone-building systems. Elevated cortisol turns "on" the fight-or-flight response and genetically reroutes both energy and micronutrients from bone-building to the muscles.

DHEA is slightly controversial because it has been misused to solely enhance athletic performance, prompting the International Olympic Committee (IOC) to ban it. Yet DHEA has a number of effects that are critical in a comprehensive bone-building plan. Low DHEA-S levels indicate a faltering adaptation response to stress and increased susceptibility to osteoporosis, loose teeth, reduced energy, electrolyte imbalances, high blood pressure, depression, cognitive dysfunction, diabetes, and accelerated aging. Consequently, low bloodstream levels of DHEA-S impact the most basic cellular functions, including irregularities in daily bone-repair functions.

Melatonin: Our Biological Clock

Numerous studies indicate that the hormone melatonin is critical for bone-building, delays aging, puts us into a deep regenerative sleep, and is a powerful antioxidant in the human brain, neutralizing, among other things, the effects of cell phone use. Melatonin is a powerful scavenger of free radicals (renegade and destructive cells that break down and destroy healthy cells throughout the body, including those in the bone) and prevents the activation of pro-inflammatory chemicals, which can lead to widespread systemic inflammation. Furthermore, melatonin protects mitochondria (little energy-producing factories) in bone cells and the brain from oxidative damage (when cells "rust" and wear out).

The pineal gland, a small endocrine gland located near the middle of the brain, is a biological clock that secretes melatonin in a circadian rhythm. Melatonin levels rise after sunset and blood levels peak between 1 a.m. and 4 a.m. For thousands of years we have depended on variations in light intensity to synchronize our biological clock. Darkness, through a positive feedback loop, turns melatonin production "on," and light, through a negative feedback loop, turns production "off." This ancient bidirectional system was understood by our wise grandparents: "Early to bed, early to rise makes a person healthy, wealthy, and wise."

Since 1945, the introduction of artificial light into every home threatened the proper sequencing of the pineal gland. Today, late-night television, videos, DVD movies, computers, computer games, chat lines, iPods, MySpace, iTunes, iHome, e-mail, the BlackBerry, video cell phones, e-Bay, downloading music, and shopping on-line have significantly altered our deep-sleep patterns and reduced our melatonin levels.

Dr. Samuel Hepworth reported in the January 2006 edition of the *British Medical Journal* that all cell phone exposure is capable of causing brain tumors or impaired brain function. Dr. Tsuyoshi Hondou, of Tohoku University in Japan, showed that non-users of cell phones, just like secondhand or passive smoke, cannot avoid microwave radiation in crowded public places like sports arenas, meetings, offices, restaurants, buses, or commuter trains. Recently, the *Archives of Medical Research* in 2005 and *Molecular and Cellular Biochemistry* in 2006 both proved that taking melatonin and other antioxidants can prevent the oxidative stress and free radical brain destruction caused by cell phones.

Only recently, researchers have found receptor sites for both melatonin and DHEA throughout bone-forming osteoblast cells. Both melatonin and calcitonin (a protein molecule that guides or chaperones calcium into bone structure) are elevated at nighttime following daytime bright light exposure. This suggests that nighttime is critically important to both bone-repair and bone-building.

Andropause in men, and menopause in women, are associated with lowered secretions of DHEA-S and melatonin with a consequential acceleration of bone loss. There is considerable groundbreaking evidence that both adrenal and pineal gland functions are linked to osteoporosis in men and women.

Transdermal and Sublingual DHEA and Melatonin Replacement

I highly encourage you, after 40 years of age, to consider sublingual or transdermal cream applications of DHEA and melatonin since these delivery systems ensure rapid uptake and assimilation of these two critical hormones into your blood and your bone-building cells.

DHEA and melatonin are lipophilic (fat-soluble) hormones that are absorbed effectively through the skin's fat cells (transdermal uptake) and allow for equal distribution throughout the body. If you consume them in a pill or capsule, your liver may inactivate them.

DHEA is used to prevent osteoporosis, low libido, stagnant energy, depression, and a faltering immune system. DHEA restores, renews, and reinvigorates the thymus gland, a critical center of the immune system. DHEA-S is an active neurosteroid that primes the hippocampus brain center to boost and maintain energy, mood, libido, and physical performance.

Melatonin has been used to prevent degenerative bone-repair and bone-building systems, depression, seasonal affective disorders (SAD), Parkinson's and Alzheimer's disease, and to initiate a deep-sleep pattern at night.

If your physician, through a simple blood test, determines that your DHEA-S level is low, you can use a transdermal DHEA cream made by a compounding pharmacist (15 mg once before sleep and 15 mg about 7 a.m.), or take a 25 mg capsule at the same times. Oral doses of DHEA are higher than topical transdermal doses because the liver converts some oral DHEA into inactive metabolites. You can also use effective sublingual (under the tongue) tablets that you allow to dissolve.

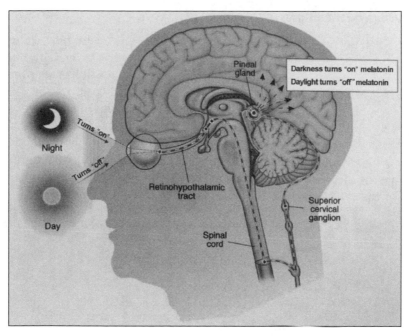

Figure 3.6: How Darkness and Daylight Affect Production of Melatonin

Source: Adapted from Leonard A. Wisneski, M.D., and Lucy Anderson, M.S.W., *The Scientific Basis of Integrative Medicine*: CRC Press, 2005.

You may use transdermal melatonin cream (3 mg applied before bedtime), or take 1–3 mg orally or 500 mcg sublingually one hour before bedtime. You will benefit more from transdermal and sublingual application than from oral capsules. The transdermal creams are applied to any soft-tissue area of the body such as the inner thighs, inner biceps, inner wrists, belly, face, and neck. Sublingual application is equal to transdermal delivery systems.

Note: 7-kito DHEA (a metabolite of DHEA) does not convert to estrogen or testosterone, but does boost bone-building and immune functions and helps to reduce body fat. You may choose to use a combination of one-half DHEA and one-half 7-kito DHEA. It is imperative that you work closely with your physician and a pharmacist in preparing these sublingual or transdermal creams or capsules. Use only pharmaceutical-grade, natural, bioidentical hormones made by an experienced compounding pharmacist under the supervision of a knowledgeable physician who understands *hormone restorative therapy* based on the results of your specific blood tests.

All of these recommendations should be followed only until saliva or bloodstream hormone levels are restored to normal levels as determined by the results of your saliva or blood tests.

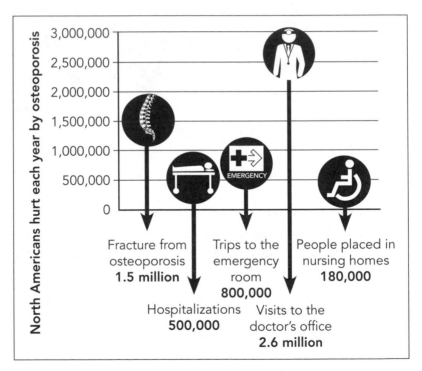

Figure 3.7: Poor Bone Health Is Common and Costly
Source: The 2004 Surgeon General's Report on Bone Health and Osteoporosis.

2000 TO 2010: THE UNITED NATIONS' "BONE AND JOINT DECADE"

The human skeleton is the single largest, living organ system, by weight, in the body. Millions of adults around the world have neglected their bone health. The problem has become so important, in fact, that the decade between 2000 and 2010 has been designated as the "Bone and Joint Decade" by the United Nations and the World Health Organization to encourage research into the "silent epidemic" of musculoskeletal, bone structure, and bio-mechanical disorders worldwide. The recognition is also designed to reinforce awareness that we must understand the many ways in which bone structure and function are affected by genetics, growth, aging, the environment, stress, exercise, diet, and a bone-building supplement.

There is now general acceptance of the importance of achieving adequate calcium (and other super-critical micronutrient) intake throughout life. For most adults, this requires using some form of "targeted" bone-building supplement daily.

Because of the intense research in this decade related to both bone and joint quality, there has been a renewed interest in research on vitamin D3. Dr. Cedric Garland and colleagues, writing in the December 2005 edition of the *American Journal of Public Health*, have shown that 800–1,000 IU of vitamin D3, taken daily, may help lower the risk of cancers of the breast, colon, and ovary by up to an astonishing 50 percent.

Recent research has also determined that your long-term bone, heart, posture, stature, fluid biomechanical movement, teeth, and nail health depends on making specific adjustments in your daily menu and supple-ment choices, most notably by daily incorporating a wider range of brightly colored fresh produce into your menu. The power of many brightly colored, healing foods comes from their broad-based ability to readily supply profound nutritional fortification for your bones' diverse biochemical processes—and protect your 100 trillion delicate cells from degenerative disease.

ADJUST YOUR GENETIC BIOCHEMISTRY

Polymorphisms (meaning many shapes) are genetic variations we have from one another, and the most common type is known as single-nucleotide polymorphisms (SNPs—pronounced "*snips*").

You can now get a genetic profile test for about $1,000, to find what SNPs you have—and determine if you are predisposed to osteoporosis—and what exact exercise, nutrient, bone-building supplement or drug, and in what quantity, you will respond positively to. Testing is done through a blood sample or mouth wash and involves 10 genetic tests to determine your exact osteoporosis risk:

- Collagen type 1 alpha 1 (COL1A1)
- Calcitonin receptor (CALCR)
- Vitamin D3 receptor (VDR)
- Interleukin-6 cytokine (IL-6)
- Tumor necrosis factor-alpha (TNF-alpha)
- Parathyroid hormone receptor (PTHR)
- Vitamin K as apolipoprotein E (APOE)
- Estrogen (ER gene) for women
- Free Testosterone (FT gene) for men
- Homocysteine (MTHFR)

Keeping your bones healthy will always be a "*present time*" challenge.

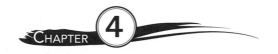

CHAPTER 4

Three Breakthrough Bone-Building Solutions

SOLUTION 1
ANCIENT WISDOM "EAT YOUR GREENS": HEALTHY BONES, HEALTHY LIFE, HEALTHY YOU!

Osteoporosis and unhealthy bones are more rampant in affluent countries than in poorer countries that still eat a lot of natural green color-coded foods. In 2005, the rural Chinese population had only 15 percent of the osteoporosis rates of wealthy North America or Europe.

When you eat any green color-coded food like broccoli, lettuce, parsley, or a "green drink" that has gone through the miracle of photosynthesis (making our vital oxygen as a waste product and consuming our deadly, exhaled carbon dioxide as a fuel), you are getting, among other things, lots of vitamin K1. You should ideally consume a minimum of 120 mcg of vitamin K1 daily.

Vitamin K1, or phylloquinone, is found in any green vegetable containing the green pigment chlorophyll and its water-soluble derivative, chlorophyllin. Vitamin K1, in the presence of "friendly" probiotic bacteria in the intestines, is converted into the more biologically active form called K2, or menaquinones. K2 is found in egg yolk, butter, and fermented soy foods.

Bitter greens like dandelions, which are filled with super-critical vitamin K1, micronutrients, and phytonutrients, are revered in China, but regarded as unwanted weeds in North America.

Vitamin K2 helps the body turn "on" biological switches that activate three critical proteins—osteocalcin, calcitonin (made by the thyroid gland), and matrix G1a—in a biochemical process called gamma-carboxylation. Osteocalcin, calcitonin, and matrix G1a are calcium-binding proteins that are absolutely essential in guiding calcium into the bone-building osteoblast cells of bones, making strong bone tissues, and preventing osteoporosis.

If you do not have sufficient vitamin K2 status, calcium may deposit in soft tissues like your arteries, heart, and brain and cause strokes, heart attacks, Alzheimer's, and dementia. Vitamin K2 simultaneously reduces the risk of osteoporosis, arteriosclerosis, and memory loss.

The journal *Nutrition* quoted the Rotterdam study of 4,983 men and women, from 1990 until 2002, which emphasized that vitamin K2 helps to protect against heart disease and memory loss. The September 2003 issue of *International Journal of Oncology* revealed that treating lung cancer patients with vitamin K2 slowed the growth of cancer cells.

The main message is to eat lots of deep-green vegetables, parsley, cilantro, watercress, culinary herbs, and "green drinks" daily.

VITAMIN K, A POWERHOUSE BONE-BUILDER THAT POPEYE UNDERSTOOD—DO YOU?

Vitamin K:

- Boosts the formation of healthy bones
- Helps maintain healthy bones
- Slows and may even stop bone loss
- Speeds up the healing of fractures
- Helps maintain the membranes of our cells
- Is a major influence in blood clotting
- Aids in fat synthesis

The body also makes its own vitamin K2. It is manufactured by bacteria in the small intestine, and because antibiotics can kill those bacteria, many researchers feel that this explains the connection between antibiotic use and damage to our bones. If you have been taking antibiotics for an extended period of time, you might want to discuss this potential problem with your doctor. It is also interesting to note that a large-scale study published in the July 2004 journal *Canadian Family Physician* found that women who received more than 100 mcg of vitamin K1 a day were almost one third less likely to fracture a hip than those who had less vitamin K1 in their diet.

The ancient, "cell-friendly" foods that are color-coded green are the richest source of vitamin K. Until recently, vitamin K had been seen strictly as a pro-clotting factor. We now know that vitamin K is the only vitamin shown to keep calcium from going into and hardening in arteries, and that it chaperones or guides calcium into the matrix of the bone.

Here are some recent research findings:

1. Dr. Richard Wood published research in December 2002 in the *American Journal of Clinical Nutrition* demonstrating that vitamin K2 boosts the gamma-carboxylation of various bone-building proteins that chaperone and deposit calcium in bones, and stops calcium from depositing as coronary plaque in our arteries causing heart attacks.

2. The *Journal of the American College of Cardiology*, in 2000, stated that suboptimal levels of vitamin K2 raised the risk of heart attacks 2.4 times—as much as smoking.

3. In 2003 the *American Journal of Clinical Nutrition* proved that vitamin K2 increased levels of and biologically upregulated the proteins osteocalcin, calcitonin, and matrix G1a protein (MGP)—three powerful "chaperones" escorting dietary calcium ions into cyclic bone-building—ratcheting up healthy bone-building all life long.

4. In August 2005 the journal *Nutritional Review* printed research that vitamin K was important in healthy bone-building function of young girls aged three to 16 years.

5. In August 2005 the *American Journal of Health Systems Pharmacology* concluded that vitamin K2 prevented weak bones, osteoporosis, and arterial calcification.

6. A Harvard Medical School study, published in the April 2005 edition of *Clinical Calcium*, demonstrated the efficacy of vitamin K2 to prevent bone loss and reduce the rate of vertebral fractures.

7. In January 2006 the *Archives of Internal Medicine* proved that warfarin (Coumadin), an anti-coagulant drug that works by interfering with the role of vitamin K2 in blood clotting (when used for more than a year) led to a 25 percent increased risk in overall fractures; a 240 percent increased risk in vertebral fractures; and a 160 percent increased risk in rib fractures.

The Story of Vitamin K and Strong Bone Development at Any Age

Vitamin K1	from green cholorphyll-rich plant foods
Vitamin K2	probiotic bacteria in the intestines convert K1 to K2
Vitamin K3	K2 converts to K3 by hydrogenated oils
	K2 converts to K3 by trans fatty acids
	K2 converts to K3 by acrylamides (fried starches, like french fries and potato chips)
	produces a renegade free radical destructive storm
	replaces K2 in the body and downregulates K2 effectiveness; vitamin K3, dihydrophylloquinone, is destructive to bone-building
Vitamin K2	turns "on" osteogenic growth levels that ignite carboxylation of calcium-controlling proteins, such as calcitonin, G1a, and osteocalcin, which chaperone calcium into bones
Strong Bones=	K2 + calcium + color-coded polyphenols + DHEA + estrogen (women) or testosterone (men) + micronutrient minerals and super-critical cofactors

The Rules of Ancient Vitamin K and Super-Critical Calcium Regulation

- Vitamin K1 is a fat-soluble (lipophilic) nutrient and is not stored in our bodies.

- The source is rich-green leafy veggies or "green drinks" that also increase polyphenols and alkalinity, reducing corrosive acidity and lowering elevated cortisol stress hormone levels.

- Osteoporosis and artery disease (heart disease and stroke) are known to be epidemiologically related; one comes with the other as both have a common basis—low vitamin K2 levels.

- With sufficient K2, calcium (Ca^{2+}) as free bloodstream calcium will deposit in bones. With low-level K2, calcium will deposit in soft tissues (such as kidneys, lungs, and brain cells), and in the interior of arterial or vascular blood vessel walls in the heart, organs, and glands.

- Low levels of inherited lipoprotein apoE4 gene + low vitamin K2 + inflammation + beta amyloid (gooey glycation) + oxidative stress = Alzheimer's disease and mental dementia.

- K2 ultimately ignites proteins to chaperone calcium into bones and out of soft tissues. Neither calcium nor vitamin D3 can produce healthy bone without K1.

Richard Wood, Ph.D., of Tufts University, who directs the Mineral Bioavailability Lab at the USDA Human Nutrition Center on Aging, reported in the December 2002 issue of the *American Journal of Clinical Nutrition* that vitamin K is a limiting factor in the gamma-carboxylation of various bone-regulating proteins.

Dr. Wood's research demonstrates that vitamin K2 is a cofactor in the chemical reaction that adds the carboxyl group (COOH) to glutamate (carboxylation), making it possible for bone-regulating proteins such as osteocalcin, matrix G1a protein (gamma-carboxyglutamate called MGP), and the thyroid-released hormone, calcitonin, to bind calcium. MGP, when properly carboxylated, is a potent inhibitor of soft tissue calcification. Dr. Wood points out that a substantial part of the North American population is deficient in vitamin K.

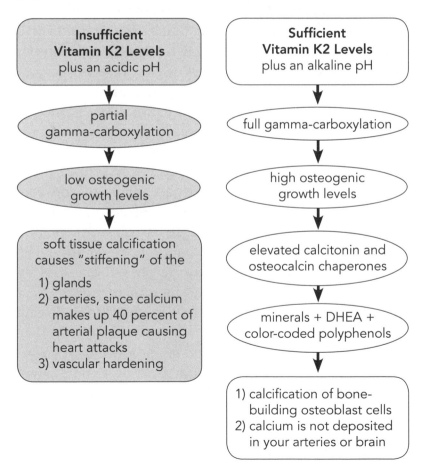

SOLUTION 2
WHY GRANDMA AND GRANDPA NEVER EXPERIENCED OSTEOPOROSIS

Just as with heart disease, the underlying rise in the "silent epidemic" of osteoporosis after menopause or andropause may *not* be primarily due to a lack of estrogen or testosterone. Although bioidentical hormone replacement therapy (BHRT) can slow the loss of bone that leads to debilitating spine curvatures and hip fractures, hormones only delay the process and can't fix it. Physicians have long known that corticosteroids will induce rapid bone loss. Well, it turns out that another mediator of the development of osteoporosis is overproduction of pro-inflammatory prostaglandlins 2 (PGE2), leukotrienes, and cytokines—"bad" types of prohormones. These system-wide communication prohormones encourage overstimulation of the osteoclast (bone-breakdown) cells, leading to weak, porous bones.

Dr. Bruce Wadkins, at Purdue University, and Professor Bruce Holub, Ph.D., of the University of Guelph, have demonstrated that high-dose fish oil supplementation rich in "mood-smart" EPA and "bone-smart" DHA has the ability to significantly decrease bone loss by decreasing PGE2 levels. Another method to reduce PGE2 overproduction is to reduce stress in your life (reducing the stress hormone levels of cortisol) and to stabilize insulin levels (since stable blood sugar levels lower your body's production of excess cortisol) by eating fewer sugars and sweetened foods. You can further reduce PGE2 by becoming alkaline.

Your grandparents' bones didn't turn to dust, probably because their diet was similar to the current recommendations in this book. They used cod liver oil instead of pharmaceutical-grade fish oil, and ate lots of green vitamin K1-rich foods, consumed fermented foods to convert K1 to its biologically active form K2, got natural sunshine on their skin (producing sufficient amounts of vitamin D3), and they walked daily and did manual chores that challenged their bones to adapt by becoming stronger. They also ate a micronutrient diet full of critical, alkalinizing calcium, magnesium, sodium, potassium, and bone-building cofactors. Their diets did not contain all the processed foods—the foods of modern commerce—that make our modern-day diets far too acidifying, which leaches calcium or potassium from the bones to buffer or neutralize the overproduction of acids by acting as acid sponges, leaving weak, porous bones.

THE DANGERS OF ACIDIFICATION: DISSOLVING CRITICAL BACKBONES

Our Bones and pH

To give you a clearer understanding of why your teeth, nails, and bones become weak and brittle from the age of 24 onward, we need to understand the dangers of acidification.

When we consume processed, fast, convenient foods and forgo our traditional salads, vegetables, fruits, berries, whole grains, and the recent addition of "green drinks," our bodies' biochemical processes become exposed; they are "under siege" by dangerous acidification.

To counter the potential, modern-day physical destruction caused by repeatedly consuming caustic, acid-forming foods, your bones break down and dissolve, releasing calcium, potassium, and sodium from the bone matrix to form chemical buffers or anti-acids called bicarbonates to soak up and neutralize the acids. The result: weak bones, poor tooth enamel quality, brittle nails, kidney stones, cardiovascular disease, heart disease, and a dissolving backbone.

The American Heart Association and the three biggest beverage manufacturers—Coke, Pepsi, and Cadbury Schweppes—on May 10, 2006 announced an agreement to take all acidifying, high-calorie, sugary drinks out of elementary school vending machines beginning immediately and progressing through to 2009. These three manufacturers have voluntarily agreed to replace these acidifying sugary drinks, which escalate the epidemic of type 2 diabetes in young people, with bottled water, unsweetened fruit juices, and low-fat milk—all served in smaller portions. And that's only the first move in this campaign to fight high-calorie foods that cause obesity and an acidifying system that dissolves our young people's tooth enamel and strong bone mass. They are planning to turn their attention next to vending-machine snack foods and fast-food companies to reduce the acidifying fat, sugar, and salt in these foods and to even outright replace them with healthier snacks.

It's Time for Healthier Alkalinizing Hospital Food

Nutritionists have started to address the incongruity of a medical establishment that bemoans obesity-related, acidifying, processed food, yet contracts with burger, doughnut, and pizza franchises for its cafeterias and loads its vending machines with chocolate bars, chips, pop, and cookies. Health-minded groups have launched movements to serve patients fresh, alkalinizing seasonal produce, and hospitals are beginning to change their

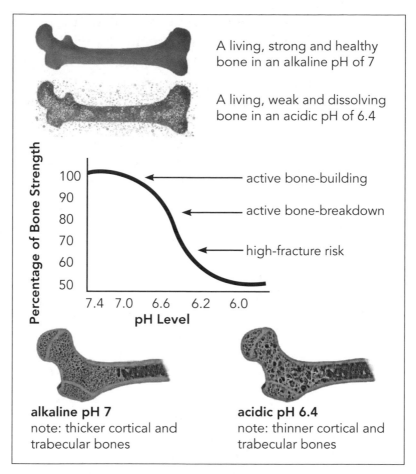

A living, strong and healthy bone in an alkaline pH of 7

A living, weak and dissolving bone in an acidic pH of 6.4

active bone-building

active bone-breakdown

high-fracture risk

alkaline pH 7
note: thicker cortical and trabecular bones

acidic pH 6.4
note: thinner cortical and trabecular bones

Figure 4.1: Bone Analysis

menus accordingly. In March 2006, Health Care Without Harm (*noharm.org*) launched a campaign for consumers such as you and I to enlist our local hospital's support.

Our Air and pH

The term "acid rain" is commonly used to describe acidic components found in rain, snow, fog, dew, or dry particles. Distilled water, which contains no carbon dioxide, has a neutral pH of 7. Unpolluted rain has an acidic pH of 5.6 because carbon dioxide and water in the air react together to form carbonic acid. However, the average rain pH today is extremely acidic with a pH between 4.2 and 4.4.

The extra acidity in rain comes from the reaction of air pollutants—primarily sulfur oxides and nitrogen oxides—with water in the air to form strong acids like sulfuric and nitric acid. The main sources of these acidic, corrosive pollutants are auto tailpipes and industrial smokestacks.

Our Soils and pH

A report published on-line January 9, 2006 by the *Proceedings of the National Academy of Sciences* explained that Duke University researchers trekked far and wide to collect soil samples from 98 locations across North and South America. To their surprise, the strongest predictor of healthy plant diversity was a neutral soil pH of 7. Acidic soils harbored only one half to one third as many natural species of plants as did the neutral pH soils. The greater the diversity in any ecosystem, the stronger is its healthy, alkaline backbone.

Our Oceans and pH

In March 2006 the prestigious magazine *Scientific American* published a feature article titled, "The Dangers of Ocean Acidification."

In 1956 Dr. Roger Revelle and Dr. Hans Seuss, geochemists at the Scripps Institution of Oceanography in California, began to measure the amount and effect of carbon dioxide spewing out of auto tailpipes and industrial smokestacks and accumulating in the atmosphere. They set up testing equipment in remote locations from

Antarctica to Hawaii to Iceland to test for high concentrations of carbon from fossil-fuel emissions.

The half-century records show that almost 50 percent of the carbon dioxide (CO_2) formed since the Industrial Revolution has ended up dissolving in all the oceans. The carbon dioxide forms into carbonic acid (H_2CO_3), shifting the oceans' natural alkaline pH of 8 to 8.3—toward worrisome acidification.

The changes in lower ocean pH chemistry are taking place rapidly, upsetting the marine ecosystem and leaving oceanic species no time to adapt. These changes are identical in consequence to the effects of acidification on the human body, causing osteoporosis and weak bone-building functions.

Acidifying oceans rich in carbonic acid make it more difficult for marine creatures to build hard, bone-like parts such as shells or coral reefs from alkaline calcium carbonate. The outcome is a globally declining ocean pH that today threatens a variety of shelled organisms like shrimp, lobster, clams, oysters, and snails, as well as coralline algae and coral reefs, which provide some of the richest habitats on earth. Acidity is causing a corrosive deteriorating quality of the ocean's corals and shells, a key link in the marine food chain.

You Are What You Eat—Ate!

Feeding cattle and cows acidifying grain can create safety issues for cattle and humans. Biologically, cattle and cows are ruminants, exquisitely evolved to graze on alkalinizing grass, and researchers have found that a grain diet raises the acidity in a steer or cow's gut. This breeds an acid resistant form of *E. coli* that can spread from feces-contaminated carcasses to meat and possibly dairy.

According to USDA researchers, more than half of all grain-fed cattle have been found to have acid resistant *E. coli* in their feces; the proportion drops to 15 percent if they are switched to grass-and hay. Beef and dairy products from 100 percent grass-fed cattle also have more conjugated linoleic acid (CLA), which recent data suggests may help prevent breast and colon cancer, as well as type 2 diabetes.

The acidifying grain-based diet contributes to one more public health problem. Overuse of antibiotics has caused more and more bacteria to become resistant to treatment, a factor in the deaths of more than 45,000 North Americans each year. An estimated 70 percent of our antibiotics (25 tonnes yearly) are fed to livestock and poultry to prevent illness and promote growth.

An acidifying grain-based diet often leads to stomach ulcers and liver abscesses in cattle and cows. Grass fed animals rarely require antibiotics. Eatwild.com is a website that links consumers to grass-fed beef and dairy ranchers. Both the American and Canadian Medical Associations have called for an end to nontherapeutic use of antibiotics in livestock.

Change the alkaline environment of Nature knowingly or unknowingly—and the new acidic environment is guaranteed to detrimentally change us! Now our human gut is far more acidic. Acid reflux disease, candida, indigestion, and malabsorption are a $9 billion dollar industry in North America alone, but it's a lot more costly than that for your health.

STAY ALKALINE TO KEEP YOUR BACKBONE STRONG

Our bodies work hard to maintain just the right level or equilibrium of alkalinity in our blood. One mechanism for correcting an excess of acidity is to dissolve some bone, releasing acid-neutralizing minerals such as potassium and calcium to form as bicarbonates in the bloodstream such as potassium bicarbonate. Potassium bicarbonate acts as an "acid sponge" to neutralize the acids in the body. This may be the main reason we experience such an escalating rate of osteoporosis in men and women in affluent Western countries.

Most amazingly, eating more alkalinizing fruit, salads, and vegetables naturally balance the acids in the body's fluids. We have a choice: By eating acidifying processed foods, we force our bones to act as large antacid tablets and we dissolve the bones' minerals to act as acid sponges. On the other hand, we can simply eat more colorful, alkalinizing produce, which naturally balance the acids and leave our skeletons intact and strong.

SOLUTION 3
A SURPRISE TOMATO ANTIOXIDANT BOOSTS BONE-BUILDING TO THE MAX

Much evidence raises the spectre that modern Western society is rife with a pernicious form of "subclinical" (symptomless) or "marginal" malnutrition that leaves no obvious traces of cellular malfunction. Your bones may get enough macrominerals, microminerals, and phytonutrients (antioxidants) to appear to function "normally." But are they really operating at optimal levels? Deteriorating bone function previously attributed to "normal aging" may, in fact, be at least partly due to subtle undetected and correctable deficiencies of specific bone-building micronutrients, say researchers from Albert Einstein College of Medicine in New York and the University of British Columbia in Vancouver.

Scientists increasingly recognize that many bone, tooth, or fracture problems from conception to death are the result of too many rampaging free radicals and not enough antioxidants. A daily firestorm of reactive oxygen (free radical) species (ROS) rip at bone cell membranes, eroding their normal functioning, and sometimes outright destroying them. You need an alert, active, surveillance-savvy police force of antioxidants, on 24-hour patrol, to limit cellular damage. You cannot avoid free radicals altogether. "Every instant of our life is an elegant and controllable dance of life and death between free radicals and antioxidants," states Montreal, Québec, pharmacist and researcher extraordinaire, Jean-Yves Dionne, M.A.

Lycopene: A Delicious Bone-Building Breakthrough

The underlying cause of miscommunication among bone cells appears to be both increased attacks by free radicals and a diminished supply of protective, micro-nutrient antioxidants (phytonutrients) from food and supplements.

Can you actually reverse bone decline? In short you can repair the bone's broken circuits, restoring most of its lost strength and functioning by consuming color-coded, "cell-friendly" foods, full of phytonutrient polyphenols and carotenoids like lycopene—a potent antioxidant. David Snowdon, M.D., of the Sanders-Brown Center on Aging at the University of Kentucky, and famous for directing the Nun Study, found that those with a "lycopene deficiency" were nearly four times more apt to require assistance than elderly subjects with above-average lycopene. Lycopene is lipophilic and enters into the bloodstream when vine-ripened tomatoes are eaten, especially when cooked with a little extra-virgin olive oil.

Although watermelon and pink grapefruit contain smidgeons of lycopene, by far the major source is tomato, notably processed tomato products, such as tomato paste and tomato sauce. A recent Italian study published in the *American Journal of Clinical Nutrition* in 1999 showed that eating tomato puree with 10.5 mg of lycopene daily for 21 days boosted the blood's antioxidant capacity dramatically. Free radical damage to cells' DNA (genetic material) dropped an astonishing 33 percent. "Daily use a bone-building supplement with 7 mg of lycopene," emphasizes renowned nutritional researcher, Professor Emeritus Venket A. Rao, Ph.D., Department of Nutritional Sciences, University of Toronto, Faculty of Medicine.

Dr. Venket Rao, Dr. Leticia Rao, and colleagues reported in August 2003, in the *Journal of Medicinal Foods*, that the red color-coded phytonutrient (carotenoid) lycopene inhibits the production of reactive oxygen species (ROS) in the osteoclast (bone-breakdown) cells, resulting in lower rates of bone-breakdown and bone loss. They concluded that, "These findings are novel and may be important in the pathogenesis, treatment and prevention of osteoporosis."

The *Asia Pacific Journal of Clinical Nutrition*, in 2003, also reported that lycopene has a positive effect on bone-building metabolism and function. The researchers concluded that, "Bone mass of the total body and lumbar spine were positively related to lycopene intake in men, and to lycopene, lutein/zeaxanthin intake in premenopausal women." The ancient and wise, color-coded lycopene neutralizes bone-depleting factors and quickly upregulates healthy bone-building metabolism and functions by acting as a powerful antioxidant in bone micro-architecture.

By the way, Dr. Snowdon also concludes, in agreement with Dr. Rao, that antioxidant lycopene in tomatoes neutralized reactive oxygen (free radical) species (ROS). As free radical damage strongly predicts a progressive loss of independence in activities of daily living, this is good news for tomato lovers!

Where to Find Bone-Building Lycopene

	1 oz Serving
Fresh tomatoes	1.5 mg
Pink grapefruit	1 mg
Spaghetti sauce	5 mg
Tomato juice	3 mg
Tomato paste	10 mg
Tomato sauce	5 mg
Tomato soup	3 mg
Tomatoes, canned	3 mg
Vegetable juice	3 mg
Watermelon	1 mg

Inarguably, good-tasting tomato antioxidants (phytonutrients) do get into our bloodstream as high circulating levels of lycopene—and into our brain, eyes, and the fatty membrane covering bone-building cells to protect their micro-architecture to eliminate destructive free radicals and antioxidant deficiencies. The results— better bones, better health, better you!

CHAPTER 5

A "Molecular-Targeted" Bone-Building Supplement

WHY SUPPLEMENT?

The vitamin and mineral content of commercially grown fruits and vegetables has declined dramatically since testing began in 1945 in both Europe and North America. In 1997 the *British Food Journal* reported research on the mineral content of fruits and vegetables grown in Europe. The research exposed for the very first time that commercially grown fruits and vegetables had their lowest levels of calcium, magnesium, zinc, and selenium since testing began.

Then, in 2002, the *Globe and Mail* newspaper in Toronto, Canada, reported new research proving that almost 80 percent of all commercially grown fruits and vegetables tested were once again at an all-time low in super-critical minerals, such as calcium and magnesium.

Finally, in 2003 the journal *Nutrition and Health* published research proving that the mineral content in commercially grown fruits and vegetables had declined drastically. Bone-building nutrients such as calcium, magnesium, copper, and zinc had by that time disappeared from our food by over 40 percent since the 1940s.

While obtaining your daily calcium requirements from food is the ideal, the fact is that almost 50 percent of North Americans' diets fall short in this regard most days of the week—or every day of the week!

It has recently been acknowledged within the scientific research community that even with a dramatic change in your diet, bone-building supplements containing calcium plus concentrated forms of bioavailable nutrients from food sources are needed to overcome the damaging effects of micronutrient deficiencies, radiation, pollution, an acidifying diet, stress, wear-and-tear, and internally generated free radicals. Micronutrient deficiencies can cause profound dysfunctions in normal cellular functioning since vitamin macronutrients, mineral micronutrients, and trace minerals are required in each of our 100 trillion cells.

Additionally, correcting micronutrient deficiencies that have accumulated over many years requires supplemental doses much greater than recommended daily intakes. Recommended daily intake levels are a guideline for healthy people and generally provide only the *minimum amount* of vitamins, minerals, trace minerals, amino acids, and phytonutrient antioxidants to prevent osteopenia or osteoporosis.

"Metabolic harmony requires an optimum intake of each micronutrient: deficiency distorts metabolism in numerous and complicated ways, many of which lead to cellular damage," states Bruce Ames, Ph.D., of the University of California at Berkeley's Department of Molecular and Cell Biology.

Harvard Medical School scientists have identified many metabolic disorders that stem from suboptimal intakes of vitamins and minerals. These researchers have stressed that supplements are not a substitute for a healthy diet, with its great diversity of phytonutrients, but should be used as a secondary therapy in preventing or treating cellular, biochemical disorders like osteopenia and osteoporosis.

> A most remarkable attribute of a properly balanced bone-building supplement is its ability to regulate cell-to-cell communication and cell-signaling activities in both the osteoblast (bone-building) and osteoclast (bone-breakdown) cells. This keeps bones strong and functional at any age.

To be effective, you must use the recommended bone-building nutritional supplement aimed at specific "molecular-targets" in the matrix of your nails, teeth, and 206 bones. A good bone-building supplement augments a healthy diet and maximizes bone-repair and bone-building functions all life long. The scientific evidence unquestionably demonstrates the benefit of a comprehensive bone-building supplement.

A comprehensive "molecular-targeted" formula boosts the bone-building osteoblast cells and ramps up sluggish osteoblast cell metabolism, which is the result of micronutrient deficiencies. Nutrients aimed at specific molecular targets in bone cells flip the bone-building switch to "on."

> Bone fractures caused by loss of bone density and strength compete with senility as the primary reason seniors are forced into nursing homes.

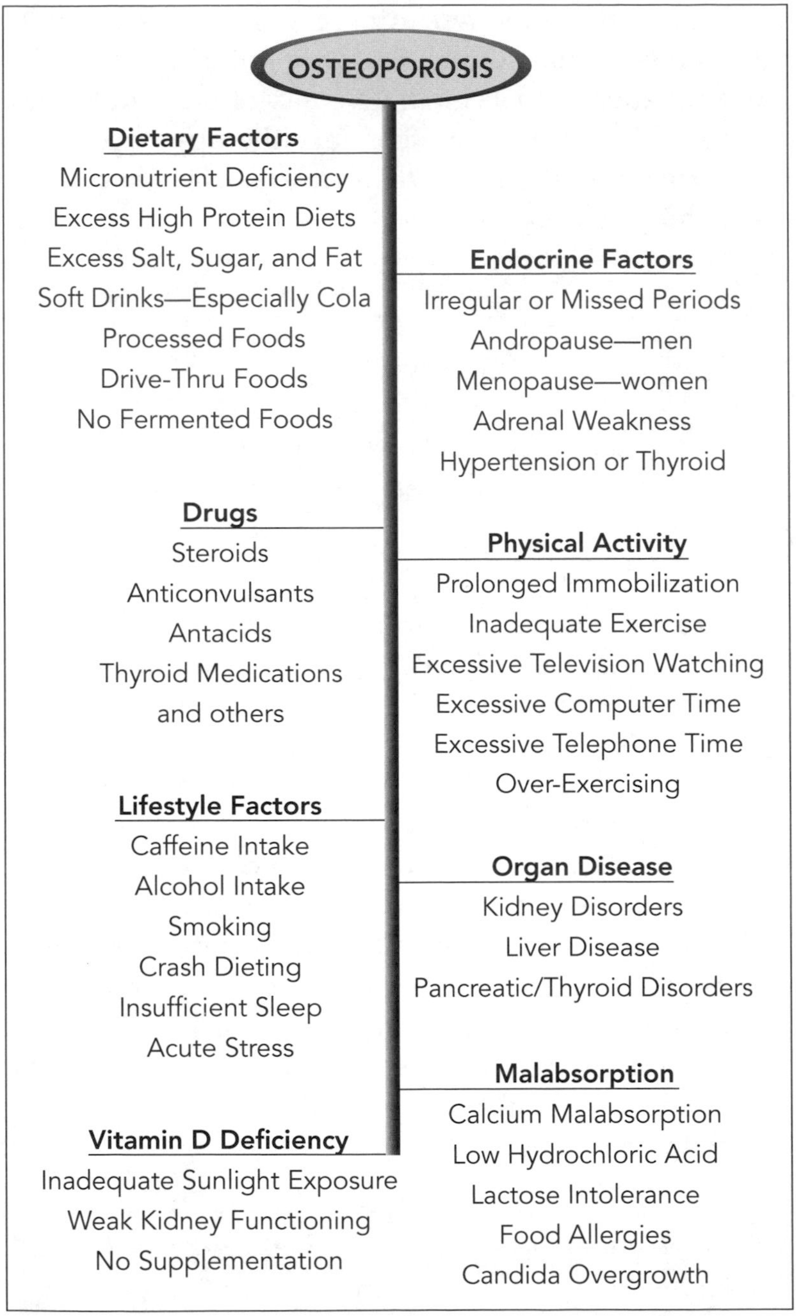

OSTEOPOROSIS

Dietary Factors

Micronutrient Deficiency

Excess High Protein Diets

Excess Salt, Sugar, and Fat

Soft Drinks—Especially Cola

Processed Foods

Drive-Thru Foods

No Fermented Foods

Endocrine Factors

Irregular or Missed Periods

Andropause—men

Menopause—women

Adrenal Weakness

Hypertension or Thyroid

Drugs

Steroids

Anticonvulsants

Antacids

Thyroid Medications

and others

Physical Activity

Prolonged Immobilization

Inadequate Exercise

Excessive Television Watching

Excessive Computer Time

Excessive Telephone Time

Over-Exercising

Lifestyle Factors

Caffeine Intake

Alcohol Intake

Smoking

Crash Dieting

Insufficient Sleep

Acute Stress

Organ Disease

Kidney Disorders

Liver Disease

Pancreatic/Thyroid Disorders

Vitamin D Deficiency

Inadequate Sunlight Exposure

Weak Kidney Functioning

No Supplementation

Malabsorption

Calcium Malabsorption

Low Hydrochloric Acid

Lactose Intolerance

Food Allergies

Candida Overgrowth

Figure 5.1: Causal Factors in Osteoporosis

Additionally, a lack of micronutrient bone-building cofactors reduces bone cells' adaptive response to stress and increases susceptibility to bone-building dysfunction and electrolyte imbalance. This results first in muscle weakness and cramping, then eventually deterioration of bone, structure, posture, fluid biomechanical movement, teeth, and nails. A "molecular-targeted" bone-building formula will increase insulin-like growth factor 1 (IGF-1) levels in bone cells to safely turn "on" bone-supportive genes and turn "off" bone-breakdown genes.

SUPERIOR BONE-BUILDING NEEDS MORE THAN JUST CALCIUM

While calcium by itself can prevent some bone loss, there are other super-critical minerals that must also be supplemented for long-term bone health and prevention of osteoporosis.

The hard-mass characteristic of healthy bone is formed by inorganic minerals such as calcium, magnesium, and phosphorus. This hard part of the bone is referred to as the "mineral mass."

The structural framework that holds the mineral mass in place is called the "organic bone matrix." The organic matrix is comprised of proteins like L-lysine, which require adequate amounts of calcium, magnesium, and phosphorus in order to function properly. The trace minerals zinc, boron, silicon, manganese, and copper, as well as non-acidic vitamins C, B6, B9, B12, K1, and the red polyphenol lycopene are essential cofactors for enzymes involved in the synthesis that make up the organic bone matrix and boost bone strength.

Regardless of your current bone health or osteoporosis bone fracture risk, you will benefit from implementing a daily, properly synthesized bone-building supplement.

PRENATAL AND PREADOLESCENT BONE-BUILDING

On January 7, 2006 the *Medical News Today* reported that researchers tracked the health of nearly 200 British children born from 1991 to 1992, along with the health, nutritional habits, calcium intake, and vitamin D3 intake of their mothers. The researchers followed up with health exams of those children at age nine to learn how those variables affected bone health specifically.

Children whose mothers didn't get enough calcium and vitamin D3 by taking a supplement or getting enough sunshine grew up with weaker bones, increasing their risk of osteoporosis, poor tooth enamel, and, surprisingly, type 2 diabetes, cardiovascular disease, and heart disease later in life. The *American Journal of Clinical Nutrition* reported in January 2005 on a study that tracked the effects of calcium on bone density in over 350 children ages eight to 13. The researchers found that:

- Elevated calcium intake during preadolescence could help prevent fractures, weak bone development, and osteoporosis later in life, as the pubertal growth spurt accounts for nearly 40 percent of the gain in the entire adult skeletal mass.
- Calcium requirements differed according to body size—taller individuals need more calcium daily during growth than shorter individuals.

The beneficial bone-density effects were found to be greatest in the group who supplemented with an additional 670 mg of calcium for a total of 1,500 mg daily.

The risk of developing brittle nails, loose teeth, stiff joints, aching bones, loss of fluid mobility, weak bones, and osteoporosis in old age is not inevitable. We must ensure that our children have enough daily calcium and all the other necessary cofactors to build a strong skeleton to prevent the possibility of developing these conditions in later years.

BONE-BUILDING SUPPLEMENTATION AND PMS

The *Archives of Internal Medicine* published research in June 2005 proving that adequate daily consumption of calcium and vitamin D3 lowered premenstrual syndrome (PMS) by 40 percent in women aged 27–44 years.

Dr. Elizabeth Bertone-Johnson of Brigham and Women's Hospital and Harvard Medical School said, "Our findings suggest that a high intake of calcium and vitamin D may reduce the risk of PMS. In the interim, given that calcium and vitamin D may also reduce the risk of osteoporosis and some cancers, clinicians may consider recommending these nutrients even for younger women."

BONE-BUILDING SUPPLEMENTATION AND CANCER

The *Journal of the National Cancer Institute* published research in December 2003 that showed evidence that calcium and vitamin D3 help prevent colon cancer, as well as cardiovascular and heart disease. A group of researchers from six major American research centers now report

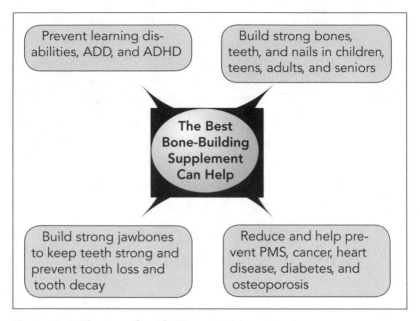

Figure 5.2: The Benefits of a Bone-Building Supplement

that a combination of a high calcium intake (providing 1,200 mg a day of elemental calcium) and a high blood level of vitamin D3 reduced, on average by 29 percent, the recurrence of colon cancer. Dr. Shin and others from Harvard Medical School, in a large prospective study based on the Nurses' Health Study database, determined that high calcium and vitamin D3 intake reduced breast cancer. This study is consistent with other studies that prove a strong association with increased intake of calcium and vitamin D3 in reduced breast cancer rates.

It's no overstatement that soybeans and soy products containing an abundance of a food polyphenol called an isoflavone have burst upon the nutritional landscape in the last few years. Recently, scientists have found a better source of isoflavones than controversial soy called *kudzu*. Two pieces of research have fueled the awareness of the potential power of isoflavones. Epidemiological studies of people who eat high amounts of isoflavones (polyphenols found not only in the soybean but also in the oriental herb *kudzu*) have surprisingly low rates of cancers of the breast and prostate.

Relatively recent research proves that isoflavones have a host of cancer-fighting properties. Like all tissues, cancerous tumors need a constant blood supply in order to survive. In men and women, isoflavones block the blood supply to cancer cells in the breast and prostate, a process known as anti-angiogenesis.

Furthermore, in women isoflavones act like plant estrogens, especially *estriol*, according to the *Journal of the National Cancer Institute* (*JNCI*). Researchers now believe that these isoflavones take up residence and bind to estrogen-receptor sites in the breasts and protect them from the cancer-promoting effects of two other estrogen fractions, *estradiol* and *estrone*.

BONE-BUILDING SUPPLEMENTATION AND HEART DISEASE

Leading researcher, Samy I. McFarlane, M.D., recently published a brilliant and impressive research paper in *Endocrine*. His exciting research suggests that there is a powerful link between osteoporosis and cardiovascular and heart disease. He writes: "Various common factors promote both vascular disease and bone loss in simultaneous fashion. Therapeutic agents in the treatment of either of these have beneficial effects on the other, suggesting common mechanisms for both diseases."

Particularly fascinating and important is that the connection between osteoporosis and heart disease, which has been a puzzling mystery of human aging, can be solved with Dr. McFarlane's research. Use a good bone-building supplement daily and you quickly reduce the rate and incidence of both osteoporosis and cardio-vascular disease in your lifetime. In a telephone interview I had with Dr. McFarlane, we mutually agreed that it is prudent to supplement daily with a food-based, bone-building supplement to build strong bones and keep calcium out of the arteries and heart where it hardens tissues, contributing to atherosclerotic plaque.

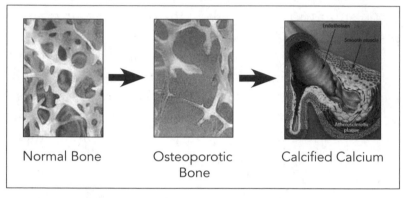

| Normal Bone | Osteoporotic Bone | Calcified Calcium |

Figure 5.3: Osteoporosis and Heart Disease Are Co-Occurring

THE ANCIENT ARCHITECTURAL WISDOM OF MINERALS

There are more than 100 separate mineral elements.

For many years, scientists focused on the role of vitamins as regulators of biochemical functions; the critical role of both minerals and trace minerals did not emerge until the late 1990s. We now understand that nails, teeth, and bones rely on specific mineral-receptor sites and cell-signaling routes for optimal uptake of minerals, trace minerals, and phytonutrients. These receptor sites are embedded deep in the micro-architecture of bone-repair and bone-building cells. Any distortion of bone architecture due to unavailable or incorrect amounts of minerals affects mineral-binding potential and alters gene-signaling expressions within each bone cell.

Here is an overview of the latest breakthrough studies published on minerals:

- Calcium and vitamin D3 reduce the risk of colon cancer, stroke, and type 2 diabetes.
- Calcium and 800 IU of vitamin D3 are powerful bone-builders.
- Calcium and vitamin D3 reduce tooth loss and brittle nails.
- Calcium and magnesium supplements improve LDL and HDL cholesterol levels in the bloodstream, reducing systemic inflammation and boosting bone-building in children, teens, women, and men.
- Suboptimal supplies of calcium, magnesium, and vitamin D3—and acidifying soft drinks—are a significant cause of type 2 diabetes in those aged 12 to 30 leading to poor teeth and weak bones.
- Zinc is critical for bone repair.
- Boron, silicon, manganese, and copper supplements reduce bone loss.
- Exercise, especially weight-resistance exercise, allows calcium and magnesium to be better absorbed by bone since bone responds to external mechanical stress.
- Lycopene, the red carotenoid (antioxidant), reduces inflammation systemically while at the same time allowing osteoblast cells to repair bone.
- Magnesium aspartate, in which most Western nations are deficient, may provide energy reserves in both chronic fatigue and fibromyalgia. Magnesium facilitates the absorption and utilization of calcium in bone-building.

Certain minerals can actually reduce the effectiveness of your bone-building supplement. Iron and calcium compete for absorption and iron always wins, so iron should never be taken in, or with, a bone-building supplement containing calcium. Strontium also competes with calcium for absorption, and it too should never be taken in, or with, calcium.

Other than the 15 essential minerals, most are non-essential and unnecessary to good health. In fact, they can represent a toxic burden to your body's elimination pathways. By competing with essential minerals for binding sites, these toxic elements can gum up your critical enzyme systems and create the same adverse health consequences that would result from a deficiency of the essential minerals. This condition is referred to as "toxic metal syndrome" and is an unavoidable feature of modern life because of the pollution that surrounds us.

In order to help maintain equilibrium in our 100 trillion cells, an optimal color-coded diet and a "targeted" bone-building supplement would supply the following essential minerals:

Calcium	Zinc	Chromium	Copper
Magnesium	Selenium	Boron	Molybdenum
Phosphorus	Manganese	Fluorine	
Potassium	Iodine	Sodium	

Iron

You notice that iron is not in the list. Iron is an essential mineral needed for the formation of hemoglobin, the molecule in your red blood cells that carries oxygen. Yet, like copper, iron is a double-edged sword. While some is good, more is not necessarily better. Both iron and copper are so-called transition metals and, under appropriate circumstances, can lead to excessive free radical production. Therefore, iron supplementation is not generally recommended because the body has no mechanism for ridding itself of excess. Some researchers have linked excess iron to heart disease, diabetes, cancer, increased mental dementia, worsening of rheumatoid arthritis, and downgrading bone-building functions.

If you do require an iron supplement, only use one under the care of a knowledgeable health care provider. Preferred sources are organic iron such as ferrous fumerate, ferrous citrate, or ferrous peptonate, usually in a dose of 300 mg. Do not use ferrous sulfate, which neutralizes and destroys vitamin E.

SUPER-CRITICAL BONE-BUILDING MINERALS

The only known natural substances to enhance bone-repair and bone-building performance are a very specific synergistic combination of both micronutrients and macronutrients that help to maintain superior bone quality in the tug-of-war between bone-building and bone-breakdown.

The best supplemental forms of minerals to take daily are those bound to small peptides, which escort or "chaperone" minerals successfully across the intestinal barrier and into the bloodstream for delivery to bones.

Minerals are critical cofactors for thousands of different metabolic enzymes. Magnesium cofactors over 350 enzymatic reactions, including those involved in heart rhythms and bone-building. Zinc cofactors over 300 enzymatic reactions, including those involved in DNA repair and bone-repair.

Below is a list of the cofactors that must be taken together to ensure superior bone-repair and bone-building at any age:

- **zinc** deficiency causes a reduction in osteoblasts, the bone-forming cells

- **manganese** deficiency inhibits organic bone matrix formation

- **copper** deficiency prevents the stable adhesion of elastin to collagen to give bone flexibility so it is strong as steel but light as wood

- **silicon** or **silica**, from the horsetail herb, is an essential nutrient for healthy bone metabolism, triggering the deposit of calcium and phosphate into bone

- **vitamin D3** is super-critical to facilitate the absorption of calcium from the intestines into the bloodstream

- **boron** helps to reduce the urinary excretion of calcium and magnesium—it preserves calcium and magnesium for bone-building

- **magnesium** can prevent migraines and is as important as calcium in healthy bone-building—the ratios can be 1.5 to 1 of calcium to magnesium

- **vitamin K2** has a direct anabolic effect on bone-building and deposits (chaperones) calcium in the bones and keeps it out of soft tissue like your heart, arteries, and brain

- **lycopene** (the red antioxidant carotenoid in tomatoes) prevents the risk of osteoporosis by reducing destructive inflammation in the microenvironment of bone

- **calcium** is critical for bone formation (your body does not absorb more than 500 mg of elemental calcium at a time)

- **vitamins B6, folic acid (B9),** and **B12** reduce systemic inflammation by reducing elevated and damaging homocysteine levels and C-reactive protein (C-RP) levels, and help to build strong bones

- **isoflavones**, vital nutrients found in high amounts in the Asian herb kudzu and fermented soy products, are related to flavonoids, which reduce the risk of hormone-dependent breast and prostate cancers and enhance bone-building.

Calcium cofactors over 250 enzymatic reactions, including the formation of critical skeletal structures. Calcium also has an important role in membrane signaling abilities and transport in the brain, and magnesium drives energy-producing reactions. Furthermore, optimum levels of calcium are associated with healthy cell membrane maintenance.

It is important to note that all minerals, except strontium and iron, should be taken together. If you take strontium and/or iron with a bone-building supplement, there is always the potential for malabsorption between competing minerals. For example, calcium should always be taken with magnesium in order to improve calcium absorption and utilization and guard against magnesium depletion, but not with strontium or iron.

WE'RE IN A CALCIUM DEFICIENCY CRISIS

Calcium is the most important mineral in your body, and the most difficult to absorb. Calcium is also the most abundant mineral in your body yet, unfortunately, people are becoming more and more deficient in it.

> It appears that too little calcium in the diet leads to decreased fat burning in cells, and therefore increases fat storage.

We are already in a calcium-deficiency crisis with 165 million people in Canada and the United States not consuming enough calcium to keep their bone-building processes operating at peak performance after their mid-twenties. Calcium, as we all know, plays an important role in maintaining healthy bones, teeth, and nails.

The average woman has about 2 lbs of calcium in her body, and the average man has almost 3 lbs in his body. One fifth of our total bone mass is calcium. About 98 percent of the calcium is stored in our bones. Another 1 percent of calcium is in our teeth, and the other 1 percent circulates in our bloodstream and tissues.

Recently the *Journal of the American College of Nutrition* reported on a new study that found people who had less calcium in their diets were more likely to gain weight than those who were eating high-calcium diets. The study recommends that it is important to get up to the recommended 1,200 mg of calcium in your diet every day. In July 2005 the *Journal of Clinical Endocrinology & Metabolism* published research that showed our total body fat is inversely related to our vitamin D3 and calcium levels. Daily consumption of low levels of calcium and less than 800 IU of vitamin D3 means more body fat.

Getting adequate calcium into your daily diet is far more important than we ever realized. The tricky thing about getting enough calcium is that it is not easy to absorb. The older we get, the harder it is for our body to efficiently absorb the calcium we give it. Yet, the older we get, the more calcium we need because our bones can lose it much faster than they did when we were younger. Nature needs calcium for structure.

Calcium is also important in weight loss. A lack of dietary calcium leads to enhanced storage of fat and a reduction in the breakdown of fat as energy. University of Colorado researchers writing in the 2003 *International Journal of Obesity* found that total dietary calcium, and not only dairy-based calcium, increased fat burning over 24 hours. Intriguingly, an additional 300 mg of calcium per day for adults was associated with 6 lbs less weight. The reason is that increased dietary calcium makes cells less likely to store fat and more likely to burn fat.

According to the National Institutes of Health (NIH), ideal calcium intake in milligrams per day should be:

Age	Optimal Calcium Intakes
Birth to six months	400 mg
Six months to a year	600 mg
1–10 years	800–1,200 mg
11–24 years	1,200–1,500 mg
25–50 (men and women)	1,000 mg
51–64 (women on HRT and men)	1,000 mg
51 plus (women not on HRT)	1,500 mg
65 and older (men and women)	1,500 mg

Note: The National Academy of Science and the Canadian and U.S. governments recommended amounts are both lower than the amounts listed above, but I prefer the higher NIH recommendations.

The NIH recommends most adults over the age of 50 should be getting 1,500 mg of calcium every day. The problem is that your body and intestines can absorb only about 500 mg of calcium at a time. Therefore, spread your calcium between your meals. Never take more than 500 mg of any calcium supplement at any one time.

The unfortunate fact is that the average adult is only getting between 200 and 600 mg of calcium a day in his or her diet. This is truly worrisome!

UNDERSTANDING CALCIUM SUPPLEMENTATION

Since the body needs between 1,000 and 1,500 mg of elemental calcium a day, the rate of mineral absorption into the bloodstream is of critical importance. The wrong form can result in a person swallowing a lot of tablets or capsules, yet absorbing very little calcium into the bloodstream and potentially causing kidney stones.

The standard high-quality calcium supplement generally contains calcium citrate as the calcium source and is superior to most commercial calcium supplements. There are three other forms of calcium that have shown far better solubility and absorption than calcium citrate. The clinically proven, most soluble and absorbable forms of calcium for human consumption are:

- calcium bisglycinate
- calcium formate
- calcium citrate-malate

Calcium lactate (from cow's milk) and calcium gluconate (a low-quality calcium source), which are highly promoted in liquid formulations, have a solubility *less* than calcium citrate! Liquid calcium supplements most often contain suspect sweeteners like artificial fructose. In animal studies, Israeli researchers discovered that eating artificial fructose may be even worse than eating sugar (sucrose or glucose). This is especially bad news because in the last few years, consumption of added fructose in foods has skyrocketed. What is new and alarming is that Dr. Roger B. McDonald, at the University of California at Davis, showed that rats fed fructose have shorter life spans than rats fed comparable calories in starchy carbohydrates. In searching for a reason, he found that sucrose, glucose, and fructose in the bloodstream react with proteins to create so-called glycated or cross-linked proteins called AGEs (advanced glycation endproducts), a cellular debris that accumulates in the brain, skin, and our 206 bones, causing bone cell DNA to malfunction. When bone cell DNA is damaged from consuming artificial fructose, it ultimately produces structural abnormalities that alter and derail lifelong calcium formation and bone-building.

Calcium and Magnesium: A Team in Bone-Building

Why Calcium Is Not Absorbed

- Magnesium, vitamin D3, and vitamin K deficiency
- Low solubility of supplemental calcium

- Low stomach acid (hypochlorhydria)
- Imbalance of cofactors
- Excess phosphorus, sugar, salt, caffeine, and pop

What Happens When Calcium Is Not Absorbed

- Calcium deposits in the arteries and joints
- Bone fractures
- Osteoporosis
- Muscle cramping in legs, restless leg syndrome
- High blood pressure
- Kidney stones or gallstones
- Brittle nails, poor teeth
- PMS, irregular periods
- Restlessness and sleep problems

Factors That Deplete Magnesium

- Excess calcium
- Acute stress and anxiety
- Excess caffeine, sugar, sodium, and processed foods

Magnesium Deficiency

- Restlessness and sleep problems
- PMS and menstrual cramps
- Muscle spasms and cramps
- Irregular heartbeat
- Headaches

Unacceptable Coral Calcium

Coral calcium has been heavily promoted to the North American public as a superior calcium source and supplement. In reviewing the materials supplied by a manufacturer, the highly regarded researchers from Life Extension of Fort Lauderdale, Florida, could not corroborate any of these claims. Coral reefs are protected by international law and hence you cannot destroy them to make coral calcium supplements. Therefore, almost all coral calcium supplements come from old, fossilized, dead coral reefs called limestone.

Limestone is also called calcium carbonate ($CaCO_3$) and it is very inexpensive. For example, you can purchase limestone wholesale for $2.00 U.S. per pound. And yet coral calcium (low-quality calcium carbonate) would cost you roughly $128.00 U.S. per pound. Coral calcium revenues from infomercial marketing and websites may account for $700 million U.S. in annual revenue in North America, according to industry estimates. All other forms of genuine, high-quality calcium supplements account for approximately $900 million U.S. in annual North American sales.

In June 2003, the Federal Trade Commission (FTC) charged the marketers of the most popular coral calcium product with making false and unsubstantiated claims about the product's health benefits. Furthermore, coral calcium has been shown to have unsafe levels of lead! Consumers are enticed by misleading information, but are unaware that they are purchasing expensive, poorly functioning, and possibly unsafe supplements. *Caveat emptor*: buyer beware is still the rule of thumb!

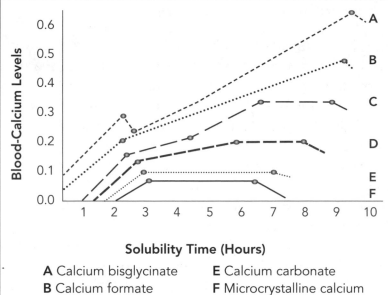

Solubility Time (Hours)

A Calcium bisglycinate   **E** Calcium carbonate
B Calcium formate   **F** Microcrystalline calcium
C Calcium citrate-malate   hydroxyapatite
D Calcium citrate
    (powder or liquid)

Note 1: Calcium bisglycinate, formate, and citrate-malate *outperform* all calciums.

Note 2: Use a calcium bone-builder formula with a maximum of 500 mg of "targeted" calcium and 300 mg of magnesium in a powdered food complex that you can simply mix with water, vegetable juice, or unsweetened fruit juice like orange juice. Magnesium supplements with more than 350 mg of magnesium can cause diarrhea.

Note 3: Liquid calcium formulations are not highly recommended because they generally contain fructose, honey, maltodextrine, and other counterproductive sweeteners.

Note 4: Calcium formate is the newest, researched, highly absorbable form of calcium.

Note 5: Microcrystalline hydroxyapatite complex (MCHC) is ground cow bones.

Figure 5.4: Calcium Solubility

THE BONE-BUILDER
SUPPLEMENT SOLUTION

Today, it is easy to follow a mineral supplement program that is scientifically substantiated to prevent and partially reverse osteoporosis. Recently, specialized multiple mineral formulas with genuine bone-building capabilities have become available.

Let's summarize what a comprehensive bone-building formula should contain.

Calcium	from citrate-malate, formate, and bisglycinate	500 mg
Magnesium	from aspartate	300 mg
Zinc	from bioactive food base	10 mg
Manganese	from bioactive food base	3 mg
Boron	from patented OsteoBoron	3 mg
Silicon	from the herb horsetail	3 mg
Copper	from HVP chelate	1 mg
Vitamin D3	natural form cholecalciferol	800 IU
L-lysine	amino acid	400 mg
Vitamin C	from non-acidic calcium ascorbate	100 mg
Lycopene	(a red antioxidant carotenoid from tomatoes)	7 mg
Vitamin B6	(pyridoxine hydrochloride)	10 mg
Vitamin B9	(folate or folic acid)	400 mcg
Selenium	from bioactive food base	100 mcg
Vitamin K1	(menatetrenone) from the "green drink" base	120 mcg
Vitamin B12	(cyanocobalamin)	10 mcg

Note: All the minerals are listed as their "elemental" dosages. For example, elemental calcium means the amount that is available to be absorbed by your body. This formula is highly absorbed in an alkalinizing "green drink" powdered base, supplying 120 mcg of vital vitamin K1 that you mix with a liquid of choice. It boosts cellular communication of bone building cells and acts as a cellular and metabolic regulator, fine-tuning bone-building composition and improving bone quality.

THE PERFECT BASE FOR A BONE-BUILDER SUPPLEMENT

The ideal delivery system for a bone-building formula is an unsweetened mineral powder mixed with quality water, or 4 oz of water plus 4 oz of an unsweetened fruit or vegetable juice. Even better, incorporate this powdered mineral formula in a symbiotic "green drink" containing a large assortment of phytonutrients such as probiotic bacterial cultures (acidophilus), prebiotics such as fructo-oligo-saccharides (to upregulate and transform vitamin K1 to the biologically active form of K2), herbs, chlorophyll, and nutrient-dense grasses like wheat grass.

Dr. Leticia Rao, Ph.D., in a research paper entitled "Polyphenols in *greens+* and Bone Health," has proven that one specific "green drink," *greens+*, all other things being equal, dramatically influenced and benefited cell-to-cell communication and active cell-signaling pathways in bones, resulting in greater bone mineral formation by osteoblasts. Her research was completed in laboratory cell lines (*in vitro*) and she plans to follow it through in humans (*in vivo*). This "green drink" is a food incorporating the ancient wisdom of color-coded eating with the most acclaimed "cell-friendly" foods. The clinically researched, food-based *greens+* enhances bone-building and bone-repair capacity, making the bone-building supplement even more uniquely effective, with both visible and tangible benefits.

All cells must receive constant positive chemical messages and optimal nutrients to live. The cell-to-cell chemical growth messengers are known as anabolic "transcription growth factors." If a bone cell does not receive daily growth factor chemical messages from bioavailable calcium and its tag team of necessary micronutrients, it will die. Brittle nails, demineralized tooth enamel, and weak bone quality are an accumulation of catabolic, derailed, and understimulated bone cells, which will develop imbalances and flaws, decrease bone-building production, and die.

The micronutrient effective formula I am presenting was designed to combine the best nutritional bone-building factors into one formulation while avoiding any negative nutrient interactions. The ultimate goal was to create a broad-spectrum blend that would effectively address bone nutritional deficiencies no matter what they may be. This formula provides 39 well-researched, bioactive, synergistic micronutrients that are carefully balanced to maximize nutritional bone structural support.

The ideal time to take a bone-building supplement is after your supper and at bedtime. Taking calcium and magnesium at bedtime can reduce restless-leg syndrome and help you get a good night's sleep.

DON'T OVERSUPPLEMENT WITH CALCIUM

The human body constantly renews osteoblasts in a process called the Age-Related Osteoblast Replicative Capacity (ARORC). If people overconsume calcium with daily intakes of 3,000 mg or more, the continuously high bone-building rates exhaust and wear out the ARORC, downregulating their capabilities to heal microfractures. More is not always better, especially when it comes to calcium supplementation. *The bone-builder breakthrough solution formula* I present to you contains 500 mg of elemental calcium. Those under the age of 50 should use it once a day, and those older than 50 should use it twice a day.

YOU ARE WHAT YOU EAT AND ABSORB!

The best supplement in the world will work only to the extent that your body is able to utilize it: We are, after all, what we absorb! From eating to absorption, your food follows a long, intricate, and potentially hazardous path through the digestive process in your small and large intestines. The digestive process breaks down your food and supplement selections into tiny molecular parts, which are then delivered through the bloodstream to your 100 trillion cells. The journal *Digestive Disorders Science* revealed that 70 percent of North American adults suffer from maldigestion, malabsorption, digestive illnesses, and unhealthy bacteria in the digestive tract.

Digestion and absorption of super-critical bone-building nutrients, for the most part, are on autopilot, controlled by delicate "friendly" probiotic bacteria and enzymes that control metabolic pathways for digestion and absorption. After spending three hours in the stomach, the digested food, called chyme, exits through the pyloric valve into the 25-ft-long small intestine, or "gut," the body's principal digestive and absorption organ.

Viable, probiotic bacteria have a powerful impact on our digestive system. If undesirable and unhealthy microbial agents such as yeast, fungus, and "bad" bacteria start to proliferate in the gastrointestinal tract from eating a suboptimal, nutrient-deficient diet, they quickly modify the intestines, triggering inflammation, cascading into compounding effects of reduced digestion and absorption—leading to leaky gut syndrome, irritable bowel syndrome (IBS), Crohn's disease, and gastro-esophageal reflux disorders.

Increased susceptibility to digestive and absorptive malfunction leads to poor bone-building, immune dysfunction, and depression from brain cells dying from malabsorption. In 2004, University of Connecticut researchers revealed that malabsorption of bone-building micronutrients led to significant bone loss in all measurable skeletal sites and, surprisingly, to a severe decline in cognitive functions leading to possible memory loss and depression. There is a gut-bone-brain connection!

Using Probiotics to Improve Absorption

The five synergistic researched and beneficial probiotics are Acidophilus (genus), Lactobacillus (genus), casei (species), plantarum (species), and Bifidobacteria (genus). The food-based "green drink" *greens+* is the ideal bone-building base as it contains all five strains of probiotic bacteria at 2.5 billion per serving in a prebiotic base called fructo-oligo-saccharides that feed the probiotics to keep them alive. The medical journal *Calcification Tissue International* published research in 2004 proving that fructo-oligo-saccharides maximize bone-building and prevent osteoporosis on their own. The probiotics in *greens+* are a therapeutic dose from non-dairy sources. These viable, probiotic strains are grown on brown rice, stabilized with vitamin C as calcium ascorbate, and freeze-dried. They are well-documented, researched strains used in medical research.

Probiotic "friendly" bacteria digest the lactose in dairy products and downgrade lactose intolerance. Ultimately, these probiotic bacterial cultures prevent unhealthy intestinal overgrowth of fungus, yeast, viruses, and "bad" bacteria that initiate or promote malabsorption of super-critical bone-building micronutrients. Without adequate probiotic levels we become susceptible to chronic fatigue syndrome, irritable bowel syndrome (IBS), fibromyalgia, the yeast overgrowth *Candida albicans*, depression, exhaustion, and porous, weak bones prone to fracture.

Antibiotics, birth control pills, cortisone, anabolic steroids, chronic constipation or diarrhea, and physical or emotional stress all quickly destroy the "friendly" and crucial probiotic bacterial cultures in the intestines.

Absorption in the intestines may be further reduced by lactic acid production and acid-resistant bacteria in an acidic colon, spurred on by eating too much dairy and sugar. D-lactate, a potentially dangerous form of lactic acid, is kept to a minimum by the activities of probiotic bacteria, which convert D-lactate into acetate and water and excrete them. An intestinal overgrowth of lactic acid, especially D-lactate, autointoxicate (re-enter) the body and accumulate in the bloodstream, bone, and brain's cells. This causes an overly acidic environment leading to depression, anxiety, and behavioral problems, spewing a potentially dangerous and antagonistic amount of inflammatory chemicals, causing accelerated bone-breakdown and bone loss.

The synergistic effect of these five probiotic strains allows the food-derived polyphenols from colorful fruits and vegetables, as well as the essential synergistic micronutrients of a bone-building supplement, to be well absorbed. This reinforces anabolic bone tissue formation and bone mineral density (BMD), therefore helping to prevent or reverse osteoporosis and thus increasing good skeletal structure, healthy posture, and fluid biomechanical movements.

LECITHIN: THE SUPPLEMENT-ABSORPTION SOLUTION

Lecithin has become a slowly vanishing crucial nutrient as Western cultures switch to low-fat diets, low-carb diets, fast-food diets, and convenient, overly processed foods. Lecithin is technically called a phosphatide complex, containing 26 percent phosphatidyl-choline. Lecithin is the most bioavailable, "cell-friendly" source of the critical B vitamin, choline. Choline is the precursor (building block) for acetylcholine, the neurotransmitter vital to encoding superior, high-fidelity memory.

Both the Institute of Medicine and the National Academy of Sciences identified choline as an essential nutrient and they recommend that adult men consume 550 mg of choline daily, women 450 mg daily, and children and teens a maximum of 1,000 mg daily. A high-quality "green drink" supplies 450 mg of choline per serving, from a food source.

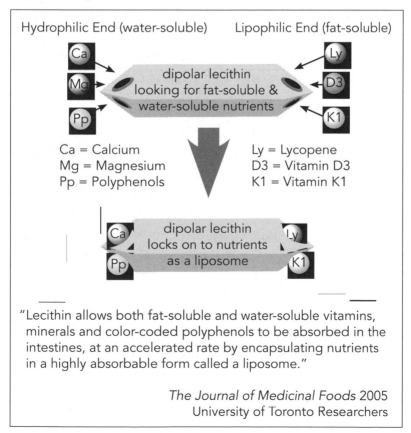

Figure 5.5: Lecithin's Unique Microencapsulation Liposome System

What researchers have further discovered about lecithin is phenomenal: One end of the lecithin molecule is *hydrophilic* (can attach water to it) and the other end is miraculously *lipophilic* (can attach fat to it). This allows your body to accelerate and vastly increase the absorption of both fat-soluble and water-soluble nutrients from food and bone-building supplements.

Lecithin also protects cell membranes from free radical damage and keeps receptor sites in the membrane soft and pliable to enhance cell-to-cell communication. Consume 2,100 mg of a phosphatide complex from lecithin daily in your bone-building supplement to boost diverse micronutrient and choline absorption, and to enhance and support superior memory and bone-building.

Lecithin, Fish Oils, and Probiotics (Halting Acute Bone Loss and Cognitive Decline)

Research strongly suggests that acute bone loss, cognitive decline, cardiovascular disease, stroke, and possibly cancer are co-occurring conditions that can be downgraded by the use of healthy probiotic cultures.

Additionally, consider taking enteric-coated fish oil capsules or liquid fish oils along with a phosphatide complex (recommended in the Product Resources section of this book). The Faculty of Medicine, National University of Singapore, proved in the January 1994 journal *Biological Trace Elemental Research* that a phosphatide complex from lecithin forms liposomes around fish oils, thus accelerating their absorption. Furthermore, these liposomes encapsulate fish oils as phospholipid liposomes and prevent lipid peroxidation (free radical breakdown) of the EPA and "bone-smart" DHA in fish oils. In September 2003 the *British Journal of Nutrition* once again proved the positive effects of lecithin on lipid (fat) absorption as lecithin induced increases in phospholipid absorption by 40 percent.

The most encouraging research comes from the University of Tromsø and Finnmark College in Alta, Norway, where researchers proved the symbiotic relationship between marine fish oils as omega-3 essential fatty acids and "friendly" probiotic bacteria. The EPA and DHA fractions of fish oils strengthen the attachment or receptor sites for "friendly" probiotic gastrointestinal bacteria, and these same probiotic bacteria (microflora) influence the accelerated rate of absorption of the EPA and DHA fractions of essential fatty acids. They concluded that, "there is a positive effect, in the normal intestine, a symbiotic relationship ... between fish polyunsaturated fatty acids and gastrointestinal bacteria strains."

Many nutritional researchers, such as Dr. Alan Logan in his highly acclaimed book, *The Brain Diet*, suggest that you have a health care provider do a lactose hydrogen breath test for you. While not 100 percent accurate, it can determine if you have unhealthy bacterial overgrowth. Dr. Logan's research also emphasizes that we should limit lactose and fructose intake and add viable probiotic bacteria to address dietary sugar intolerances and unhealthy, small intestinal bacterial overgrowth. That is why it is especially imperative to take in more healthful probiotic cultures daily to maintain a steady balance of healthy bacteria. The most recent exciting discovery—a breakthrough in understanding—is that a phosphatide complex from lecithin, healthy probiotic bacteria, and marine fish oils rich in EPA and DHA are symbiotic, facilitating each other's absorption at an accelerated rate. This also means that they reduce unhealthy bacteria in your intestines and correct maldigestion and malabsorption disorders, which are rampant in North America.

As a further example of synergistic interplay, plant lignan polyphenols from flaxseeds, are changed by the gut-friendly probiotic cultures into enterolactone and enterodiol, two compounds found to be very effective in reducing systemic inflammation and protecting against cancer, especially breast cancer. Researchers at the University of Toronto, Princess Margaret Hospital, found that women who consumed 25 g of ground flaxseed (2 tbsp) daily had a reduced risk of developing repeat breast cancer. Flaxseed lignans, ignited by probiotic cultures to become *enterolactone* and *enterodiol* (potent anti-cancer food compounds), are very beneficial for fighting breast cancer because their structure is very similar to anti-cancer drugs such as Tamoxifen and Raloxifene.

Remember that a large amount of recent research has proven that healthy probiotic cultures in the intestinal tract convert vitamin K1 into the biologically active form, vitamin K2, which is so critical for igniting small protein peptides that chaperone minerals into the micro-environment of bone-building, preventing them from forming hard, calcium-based plaque in your brain, heart, and arteries.

Nowhere is damage from malabsorption more tragic to your wellness than in your bones and brain. I recommend that you give your bones and brain a steady supply of symbiotic fish oils, lecithin, and viable probiotic cultures daily!

THE POWERFUL PHOSPHATIDE COMPLEX IN LECITHIN

Two of the most scientifically promising memory boosters are phytonutrients with tongue-twisting names: phosphatidyl-choline and phosphatidyl-serine. Most experts call them PC and PS, and Stanford University researchers showed that they dramatically restore memory loss due to normal aging. The only food source of PC and PS is a phosphatide complex from lecithin such as soy lecithin granules.

Phosphatidyl-Choline (PC)

Phosphatidyl-Choline (PC) is a phospholipid in lecithin, a large molecule that covers the fatty lipid bilayer of both brain and bone cells that ratchet up the transfer of information between cells. A lack of phospholipids can result in abnormal brain or bone communication patterns.

Phosphatidyl-Serine (PS)

Phosphatidyl-Serine (PS) helps the brain and bone cell receptors to use fuel more efficiently by boosting neuronal metabolism and stimulating production of acetylcholine in the brain. PS is able to improve the memory and brainpower of people in cognitive decline. Studies have revealed that supplementing with PC and PS slows down—and even reverses—declining memory and concentration, or age-related cognitive impairment in middle-aged and elderly subjects, according to the June 1999 journal *Alternative Medicine Review.*

PS is a phospholipid found in the outer membrane of all cells, but is most highly concentrated in the walls (membranes) of brain and bone cells, making up about 70 percent of its nerve tissue mass. PS and PC enhance the storage, release, and activity potential of many information transmitters and their cellular receptors, aiding cell-to-cell communication.

In the brain, PS and PC stimulate the release of dopamine, a mood regulator that also controls physical sensations and movement. They increase the production of acetylcholine (critical for superior learning and memory), enhance brain glucose metabolism (the actual fuel used for brain activity), reduce cortisol levels (the stress hormone), and boost the activity of brain-derived neurotrophic factor (BDNF), nerve growth factor (NGF), and neuropeptide Y (NPY), which increase the amount and health of cholinergic neurons in the brain, according to the Scandinavian medical journal *Acta Neurological Scandinavica*. Aerobic exercise and fish oils also increase BDNF, NGF, and NPY levels in your brain, boosting your brainpower.

When you supplement with: (1) a "green drink" food-based bone-building supplement rich in a phosphatide complex of choline, PC, and PS, and (2) an omega-3 fatty acid supplement from fish oils such as the clinically proven *o3mega+ 3679*™, rich in bone-building EPA and DHA, you can positively influence and increase BDNF, NGF, and NPY levels in the brain. This allows brain development of a bigger memory board and brainpower even in older adults. Therefore, smartly combining the comprehensive bone-building formula in this chapter with *o3mega+ 3679*™, which is not associated with the typical odor and fishy repeat of standard fish oil capsules, enhances your good mood, memory, brainpower, and healthy bone function for a lifetime. Together, they reduce inflammation in the microenvironment of bone.

Glyceryl-Phosphoryl-Choline (GPC)

As if the marvel and magic of a phosphatide complex from lecithin were not enough, it also contains glyceryl-phosphoryl-choline (GPC). GPC reduces arterial plaque, lowers blood pressure, and enhances memory. GPC has been shown to improve the conditions of people with adult-onset cognitive dysfunction, Alzheimer's disease, and stroke-related mental impairment. PC, PS, and GPC are available in a natural food form, piggybacking upon one another in symbiotic support, in a phosphatide complex derived from lecithin and available in the clinically proven "green drink" greens+, the perfect food base for a bone-building supplement.

According to Duke University Medical Center researchers, what is most amazing is that those parents who consume diets rich in choline, PC, and PS have offspring with brain functions that have better learning and memory capacity.

ADAPT, GROW, AND CHANGE

Our generation has been celebrated for its willingness to challenge the prevailing assumptions of society. Rather than viewing the second half of life as a time of progressive deterioration in body and mind, see aging and maturity as a time and an opportunity for greater wisdom, meaning, joy, creativity, and increased mental and physical capacity.

More people than ever before are living healthy lives into their eighties, nineties, and beyond with good bodies and bright minds. You can be one of them! You can influence your overall health, including the quality of your brain and bones, all life long through the food and supplement choices you make every single day. Unquestionably the number one aid in preventing or reversing the hazards of sore, stiff, weak bones, teeth, and joints is to use a "molecular-targeted" bone-building supplement. You will then be upgrading the real meaning of remaining healthy.

Let your body's natural wisdom point the way. You can initiate change in your life by transforming the only thing you ever had control of in the first place, which is yourself. Many men and women are now committed to optimizing and maintaining their bone-building health and well-being for as long as humanly possible. I encourage you to be among them!

A NOVEL WAY TO REGROW LOST OR BROKEN TEETH

Drs. Jie Chen and Ying Tsui, engineers at the University of Alberta in Canada, developed a miniature device that uses ultrasound stimulation to encourage damaged teeth and jawbone tissue to regrow into healthy teeth. Dr. Tarek El-Bialy, from the Faculty of Medicine, at the University of Alberta, published research in 2003 in the *American Journal of Orthodontics and Dentofacial Orthopedics*, showing that low-powered ultrasound encourages growth of dental tissue and new teeth, but only when some tooth root has remained in place.

The ultrasound device fits neatly inside a person's mouth like a brace and could help athletes, children, and adults regrow damaged teeth. Their theory is that pressure waves mimic the effect of strenuous exercise, loading a bone, and tricking it into generating more bone-building cells—a process called osteogenesis.

CHAPTER 6

The Ancient Laws of Color-Coded Eating: Solving the Bone-Building Puzzle

PART 1:
EAT A "CELL-FRIENDLY" DIET

The renowned Michael Fossel, M.D., Ph.D., Clinical Professor of Medicine at Michigan State University, said these revolutionary words to me: Think like a cell—eat a "cell-friendly" diet.

At that time I was a well-recognized Nutritional and Lifestyle Researcher. I had started a successful research company in the United States called Advanced Nutritional Research (ANR), which specialized in making cutting-edge supplements for orthomolecular physicians.

I had been fortunate to have worked with the two-time Nobel Prize winner Linus Pauling, Ph.D., "the father of vitamin C"; Dr. Zoltan Rona, M.D.; Dr. Robert Atkins; Dr. Julian Whitaker; Dr. Lester Packer; Dr. Karlis Ullis of UCLA; the renowned psychiatrist Dr. Abram Hoffer; Dr. Denham Harman, M.D., Ph.D., of the University of Nebraska, the father of the free radical theory; and two of the most dedicated and progressive promoters of superior human health in North America, William Faloon of Life Extension and Stewart Brown of Genuine Health.

Dr. Fossel's words struck me deeply and the echo kept penetrating my imagination: Eat a "cell-friendly" diet—think like a cell!

Ratchet up Genetic Bone-Building Systems in Bone Cells

Medical research agrees that our bodies' innate wisdom is undeniably found in each one of our 100 trillion cells. We are made of 100 trillion little pieces. Cells have been unconditionally supporting and out-thinking us for most of our lives—even for thousands of years.

> *Designer therapeutics*, found in colorful fruit and vegetables, send healthy "package and ship" nutrients to cells. It is like affixing a specific zipcode or mailing code onto them that guarantees exact delivery instructions to maintain and enhance healthy bone function.

When our cells are fed the *designer therapeutics* naturally found in whole, live foods, the foods' ancient genetic code turns "on" various groups of beneficial human enzymes, which trigger every biological reaction in the human body, regardless of our human genetic variations. These enzymes and coenzymes are responsible for ramping up and enhancing our cells' unfailing commitment to optimizing and maintaining our health and well-being. The precise intensity of these enzymatic, biochemical interactions is partially determined by your genetic inheritance, but your environment and lifestyle choices influence the 100 trillion cellular behaviors even more seriously. Deteriorating quality of our nails, teeth, and bones, or any physical health crises, can be surprisingly alleviated by a proper change in lifestyle, food choices, supplements, and environment.

Your 100 Trillion Cells Need Food and Nutrients Daily

Each cell in the human body works for the benefit, welfare, and health of the whole body; its individual benefit, welfare, and health come second. Individual cells will, if necessary, die to protect our bodies, and often they do. The lifetime of any one individual cell is very short compared to our own lifetime.

Every minute thousands of immune cells that fight off invading germs and toxins, facial skin cells that replenish wear-and-tear, or bone cells that repair or build become exhausted and die by the thousands. This continuous cellular renewal means that we can then lead healthier and richer lives instead of suffering from arrested development due to extreme cellular exhaustion. Cells are hardwired to know how to survive, communicate in real time over secure lines, self-repair, and create our dynamic energy supply.

Be a Co-creator to Life, Not a Victim

Although each cell, according to its individual genetic heritage, has a specific and creative set of tasks, each is flexible to adapt and respond to other immediate bio-chemical needs, anywhere in the body, with 100 percent loyalty and total effort. Each cell operates according to different rules. They are a firestorm of electrochemical

activity, never changing a single inherited communication pattern. This implies a miraculous but fragile
rhythm that must remain in precise balance since cells
are totally dependent on daily nutrient needs. Your
daily food choices manipulate, for better or worse, the
invisible forces that determine your physical health and
dictate your level of brainpower, disease resistance, and
optimum bone-building potential. This activity goes on
invisibly inside each cell and, to medical researchers,
still remains deeply mysterious.

Our cells have already revealed deep secrets. It's
worth pausing for a moment to realize that your cells
ultimately create, maintain, and drive your healthy
storyline, not you. Before 1980 medical researchers
agreed that the brain's capacity for intelligence was very
unique. In the 1980s it would have been absurd to speak
of the heart, the bones, the immune system, or the intestines as intelligent and capable of thinking.

In the 1990s a sweeping medical revolution encouraged research scientists to look into the hidden dimensions
of cells. In the late 1990s it was revealed that each cell has
intelligence and makes intelligent decisions apart from
the brain. The stomach and intestinal tract actually
think. They separate vitamins, minerals, trace minerals,
and phytonutrients from food and courier them to target
cells throughout the body with a great degree of precision.
They not only extract nutrients from food, they keep in
touch with the nutritional needs of cells in every distant
part of the body. Our stomach and intestines may be
cooperating with our entire biochemical body better
than we manage to. My father would always talk about
his "gut reaction" in making a decision or choosing
a reliable course of action he was comfortable with.
Surprisingly, Dr. Tamas L. Horvath, of the Yale School of

Medicine, has recently found that a hormone *ghrelin*, produced in the stomach, enhances learning and memory performance in the neurons of the hippocampus. The type of food you eat enters your stomach and sends "good" or "bad" learning-potential messages to your brain that turn on electrochemical activity to unite every cell in the body.

Cells Trust That We Will Fuel Them Abundantly

The immune system has surveillance outposts in every remote cell of the body, bringing information back to itself and the brain simultaneously, using special messenger molecules. The cell's wisdom is undeniably real, with astonishing, complex intelligence that is finely tuned for reacting spontaneously and reliably to both outside and internal events or stimuli.

Our cells utilize the smallest expenditure of energy to operate at their optimum level of efficiency, leaving most of our energy at our command and disposal.

Our cells function with absolute loyalty seven days a week, 24 hours a day, faithfully and trusting totally that we will provide precise nutrients and abundant fuel for them.

> Meanwhile, nutritional research continues to reveal the powerful ability of food components called phytonutrients to build or repair our bones, teeth, or nails, while downgrading and modifying potential disease processes.

The primary activity of any of our cells is to give relentlessly for our bodies' optimal benefit. To all appearances, this is how cells go about their work, day in and day out.

We need to ask ourselves if, by our very own daily poor lifestyle choices, we are starving our cells into dysfunctional activity, pain, suffering, neglect, and death. Or are we co-creating a new and wondrous quality of cellular function with wise food, supplement, and lifestyle choices?

Ancient "Cell-Friendly" Foods vs Foods of Modern-Day Commerce

Our cells must utilize the exact foods (fuels) we give them through our daily food choices. Unfortunately, today, many of our faithful cells die prematurely, searching in vain for life-saving nutrients to consume. There are no nutrients in our overly packaged and highly marketed processed, fast, or convenient "lifeless" foods. They only promote an unhealthy grab-and-feed attitude.

These are the foods of modern-day commerce. Food processors are not aware of the ancient, "cell-friendly" nutrients and color codes that foods must contain to ignite cellular, biochemical, and enzymatic processes. These foods may look good, smell good, and taste good, but, as far as our cells are concerned, they continuously fail to deliver exact natural nutrients. Cellular communications and ancient biochemical functions misfire or derail and our self-repair functions, health, and well-being are severely compromised—by our very own hands.

It's this simple: Do not deny, repress, and destroy your very own cells' critical lifeforce.

If we fuel our cells' *total activity potential*, our cells automatically respond with an immediate, healthy response. We need to feed and fuel our cells with the ancient wisdom inherent in each and every colorful fruit, berry, vegetable, sprout, salad, "green drink," herb, spice, seed, nut, whole grain, essential sea vegetable, pea, and legume. Be continually aware that the many food, supplement, and lifestyle choices we make every day are the very keys that turn "on" or "off" our optimum health, moods, happiness, quality bones, longevity, emotions, and brain functions.

Enhance Your Cells' Total Activity Potential with "Cell-Friendly" Foods

The first step is to understand the ancient wisdom in the natural food chain. Eating food is the most intimate experience we will ever have. Every food we eat becomes our hair, skin, vision, hearing, mood, memory potential, sleep pattern, creativity, immune system, heart, lungs, kidneys, libido, nails, teeth, and bones. Before you eat any meals or snacks, bless your food with gratitude and appreciation.

Look at your potential food choices and ask yourself, "Do I want this food to become my facial skin, my hair, brain, or bones?"—because it will. Live, choose, and eat wisely in harmony with your long-standing genetic predisposition to natural, nutrient-dense foods.

Bone Cells + Healthy Food Choices = Miraculous Alchemy

These simple, powerful upgrades and makeovers to your diet are completely natural and within your reach. Healthy foods are full of well-known bioactive ingredients that provide ultimate nutritional support for every cell and immediately address accumulated nutritional deficiencies, no matter what they may be.

Think like a cell! Feed your faithful and selfless cells carefully, wisely, and effectively with a broad-spectrum blend of colorful, "cell-friendly" foods. These nutrient-dense foods give all your cells sustenance and strength to overcome disease, illness, and environmental assaults. You then feel secure, trusting your own body's internal wisdom. And there is even greater magic at work. At the subatomic chemical level, nutrient-dense foods suddenly and spontaneously break down into new and crucial components that perform a feat of alchemy, preserving and supporting the orderliness of our lives while allowing diverse chemical processes to buzz, zigzag, and swirl around each cell in apparent chaos at close to 150 mph.

> It takes more moxie to adapt to reality than to avoid it.

Packaged, Shipped, and Delivered by Courier

Most research results clearly show that the average North American has significant subclinical micronutrient deficiencies and imbalances, causing cells to lose their competitive drive and resulting in daytime fatigue, poor libido and stamina, allergies, arthritis, obesity, diabetes, immune suppression, and the growing "silent epidemic" of osteoporosis, even in young people. Research scientists suggest that a simple, appropriate remedy to reset the balance between suboptimal anabolic (building) and catabolic (breakdown) metabolic disorders in the body is to eat more "cell-friendly" foods.

The power of healing in "cell-friendly" foods comes from their broad-based ability to prevent disease by nutritionally fortifying the biochemical processes that have been naturally selected by "genetic predisposition" to protect us from illness, disease, and accelerated aging.

The latest research proves that colorful, "cell-friendly" foods are necessary for long-term health and that their colorful phytonutrients (disease-fighting compounds) act as antioxidants.

1. *Proanthocyanins* give all berries (raspberries to blackberries) their pigmented colors and in 2004, Johns Hopkins reported that proanthocyanins suppressed pain caused by inflammation as much as the pain-relief drugs ibuprofen, naproxen, and Indocin®. Furthermore, fish oil supplements rich in EPA and DHA also reduced inflammation.

2. *Salvestrols (resveratrol)* in dry red wine made from cabernet sauvignon grapes (one glass per day) reach the brain within minutes and reduce the risk of Alzheimer's by 70 percent, according to the *European Journal of Epidemiology* in April 2000. Furthermore, the journal *Archives of Neurology* reports that eating dark plums, also rich in salvestrols, reduced the risk of Parkinson's disease by 76 percent.

3. *Solanine* in green vegetables inhibits the enzyme acetylcholinesterase from breaking down. This enzyme is crucial for relaying cell-to-cell messages quickly in the brain and is necessary for good memory, quick learning, and sheer brainpower.

4. Semisweet dark chocolate (70 percent cocoa or more) raises levels of two critical "feel good" hormones—serotonin and beta endorphins—and the "I'm energized" hormone dopamine. Dark chocolate contains many beneficial antioxidants.

5. The color-coded red carotenoid pigment, lycopene, neutralizes and blocks fat-related oxygen free radical species, such as those that damage good cholesterol called high-density lipoproteins (HDL), and protects bone membrane micro-architecture from structurally damaging free radical assaults.

6. In 2005 the journals *Nutritional Neuroscience*, *Experimental Neurology*, and *Neurobiology of Aging*, all reported that phytonutrients from spirulina, spinach, and blueberries do indeed cross the blood-brain barrier and protect healthy brain and bone functions as antioxidants. Documented evidence from these studies conclude that:

   • spirulina phytonutrients are quickly absorbed and act as powerful, system-wide antioxidants protecting cell membrane integrity in the brain, central nervous system, and bone membrane micro-architecture

   • bilberry antioxidants combat a range of eye disorders

   • bilberry phytonutrients protect against glaucoma by supporting healthy intraocular pressure

   • the red carotenoid, lycopene, has powerful antioxidant protection for the fatty cellular membranes on bone-building cells and in the brain

   • blueberries increase auditory processing speed by 50 percent

   • pterostilbene, a phytonutrient in all dark pigmented fruit or berries, lowers cholesterol and reduces heart disease.

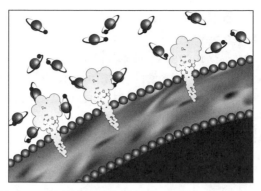

Figure 6.1: Renegade Free Radicals Hit and Tear at Bone Cells

Troublesome free radical renegades hit and tear at cell membranes, proteins, and DNA at an estimated rate of 100,000 hits a day. This free radical storm causes the wear-and-tear you see in your skin, hair, robust vitality, memory, diminishing brainpower, balance, stature, posture, fluid biomechanical movements, brittle nails, failing tooth enamel, and derailed bone-building.

This damage begins showing up by age 24, is measurable at 34, and continues to damage cells quietly, cumulatively, and without any warning symptoms all life long. Antioxidant phytonutrients (polyphenols) from "cell-friendly" colorful produce and supplements deactivate and de-energize free radicals.

You are now ready to begin a new day, in a new life of awareness and mastery. I hope this book will bring you both!

PART 2:
THE LAWS OF ANCIENT
COLOR-CODED EATING

Changing how you feed your cells and bones is the best way to quickly improve your health, and it's the easiest thing to do.

Brightly colored foods contain a huge variety of minerals, trace minerals, vitamins, antioxidants, beneficial food components, and phytonutrients to improve your bone health, energy levels, memory skills, and good mood consistently and dramatically. They are also more satisfying compared to their processed counterparts, which shorten your life span and weaken your bones, teeth, nails, and cardiovascular health.

Phytonutrients are plant pigments that give a plant its distinctive bright color and also possess potent disease-fighting properties. *Phyto* is a Greek derivative that means "from plants." Plants that have similar colors have related disease-fighting properties.

When you correctly choose foods for their vital and varied colors, you avail yourself of these healing food components or natural food chemicals. Each color has a formidable array of specific vitamins, minerals, trace minerals, antioxidants, and enzymes to improve cellular metabolism. They modify or turn "off" diseases and give your 100 trillion cells repair and restorative properties.

Why Some Foods Are Critically Important throughout Your Lifetime

Phytonutrients are made up of many subgroups or categories with diverse chemical structures, tongue-twisting names, and nutritional components that determine their color, smell, taste, and binding affinity in cells, tissues, glands, and organs. Plants make both water-soluble (hydrophilic) and fat-soluble (lipophilic) phytonutrients to act as antioxidants to protect themselves. Since the 1990s, numerous studies have confirmed that phytonutrient deficiencies impair the immune system, leading to more colds and infections, as well as weak bones, poor tooth enamel quality, and brittle nails.

Remember, the core of growth and change is to risk challenging the negative perception of fresh fruits and vegetables we have accepted from our childhood.

Phytonutrients are the buzz among food scientists because these ancient, powerful, and amazing natural plant pigments have been proven to prevent many cancers, inflammation, depression, Alzheimer's, and premature aging while boosting dramatically bone-repair and bone-building properties.

Andreas Constantinou, Ph.D., from the University of Illinois-Chicago, specializes in foods and cancer prevention. Remarkably, Dr. Constantinou found that a subclass of phytonutrients called polyphenol compounds contain ellagic acid and salvestrols, which inhibit the enzymes responsible for damaging DNA replication and initiating some forms of cancer.

Ellagic acid and salvestrols are found abundantly in blackberries, blueberries, raspberries, strawberries, beets, dry red wine, curries, ginger, and red apples. Ellagic acid and salvestrols modify genetic architecture by turning "off" genetic switches, putting the brakes on the initiation or promotion of many cancer cell colonies. It appears that this ancient wisdom inherent in colorful plants was well understood by our wise grandparents, who proclaimed, "An apple a day keeps the doctor away."

A shocking 70 percent of the foods we eat today are processed—the foods of modern commerce. In 1956 only 10 percent of the foods we ate were processed.

Apples: A Simple, Bare-Bones Solution

Dr. Stuart Silverman, a clinical professor of medicine at UCLA, said, "Right now, osteoporosis is under-recognized, underdiagnosed, and undertreated." He said we should eat apples—yes—apples. New research from the University of Massachusetts Lowell and from Saint Genes-Champanelle, France, show that apples are healthy bone-builders in both men and women.

Despite their relatively high sugar levels, apples actually exert a stabilizing effect on blood sugar, thanks in part to their high fiber content, but also because they contain *phloretin*, a polyphenol (phyto-nutrient), blood sugar-stabilizing compound found exclusively in apples. Apple peels are the potent, con-centrated source of phloretin, which is already creating some head-turning findings.

Incredibly, our bones are greatly influenced by what we eat. Phloretin increases bone-building, boosts bone mineral density (BMD), and slows down and con-trols the breakdown rate of bone (bone resorption or bone remodeling).

What Are the Ancient Color Codes?

A diet rich in colorful fruits, berries, vegetables, "green drinks," herbs, and spices improves bone metabolism and maximizes bone health, which is a real concern for men and women 34 or older.

Recent research has shown that the individual color of foods have specific health benefits. On a daily basis we should try to consume a wider variety of colors in our fruit and vegetable choices. Without the entire tag team or complement of a rainbow of colors in your daily diet, some waste materials, toxins, and free radicals will not be neutralized and will accumulate in your body, causing faulty biochemical processes. The rule of all ancient color-coded foods is that the phytonutrients in each color ride piggyback on each other and ultimately work as powerful bone-building inducers and immune system modulators. They all have a collective affinity for cellular membranes. As membrane antioxidants they maintain membrane fluidity and improve intercellular communication pathways. They work as a cellular anti-freeze and protect cells from environmental stress.

There are six main color-coded groups with several prominent phytonutrients in each group.

1. *Green:* indols, isothiocyanates, sulphoraphane, quercetin, sulfur, apigenin, glucosinolates, solanine, polyphenols, chlorophyll, chlorophyllin, thiosulfo-nate, diindolylmethane, isoflavones

2. *Red, orange, yellow:* alpha-, beta-, delta-, and gamma-carotenes, lycopene, xanthones, proanthocyanins

3. *Light to dark brown:* phytosterols, salvestrols, saponins, phytoestrogens, kaempferol

4. *Black, blue, purple:* flavonoids, proanthocyanins, pterostilbene, resveratrol, salvestrols

5. *White to golden:* omega-3, omega-6, omega-7, and omega-9 essential fatty acids

6. *Bright yellow:* astaxanthin, canthaxanthin, lutein, zea-xanthin, phytofluene, luteolin, phosphatidyl-choline (PC), and phosphatidyl-serine (PS)

Green Color-Coded Foods

Cruciferous Vegetables	Garlic Group	Mustard Vegetables	Onion Group	Herbs, Spices, and Tea
asparagus	garlic	arugula	all onions	green tea
bok choy	sprouts	daikon	chives	matcha green
broccoli		horseradish	green onions	peppermint
broccoli sprouts		mustard greens	leeks	spearmint
brussels sprouts		radishes	scallions	
cabbage		sprouts	shallots	
cauliflower		wasabi		
collards				
dandelions				
kale				
lettuce				
parsley				
rapini				
watercress				

Orange, Red, and Yellow Color-Coded Foods

Fruit	Vegetables	Herbs and Spices
apricots	beans	cardamom
apples	beets	cayenne
bananas	carrots	cinnamon
cherries (tart)	corn	curry

Fruit	Vegetables	Herbs and Spices
cantaloupe	lettuce	ginger
grapefruit	red chillies	nutmeg
lemons	squash	saffron
mangoes	sweet peppers	turmeric
mangosteen	sweet potatoes	
nectarines	tomatoes	
oranges	yams	
papaya		
pineapples		
pomegranates		
raspberries		
strawberries		
tangerines		

Blue, Purple, and Black Color-Coded Foods

Fruit	Vegetables	Herbs, Spices, and Tea
acai cherries	beans	all dark herbs
apples	blue corn	allspice
blackberries	eggplant	black coffee
black cherries	Japanese purple potato	cocoa
blueberries	peppers	curries
boysenberries	radicchio	dark chocolate
sour cherries		dry red wine
cranberries		black tea
currants		
grapes		
plums		
pomegranates		
prunes		

Light to Dark Brown Color-Coded Foods

Grains	Legumes	Nuts and Seeds	Vegetables
barley	all beans	almonds	*mushrooms:*
brown rice	chickpeas	Brazil nuts	cordyceps maitake reishi
buckwheat	edamame	cashews	
bulgur	lentils	coconuts	shiitake
millet	miso	flaxseeds	portabella
oats	soybeans	hemp seeds	
rye	split peas	macadamia nuts	*yeast:*
whole wheat	tempeh	peanuts	saccharomyces
	tofu	sesame seeds	
		sunflower seeds	
		walnuts	

White to Golden Color-Coded Foods

Fish Oils	Vegetable Oils	Protein
long-chain omega-3 essential fatty acids rich in "mood-smart" EPA and "bone-smart" DHA	*short-chain omega-3 essential fatty acids:* flaxseeds hemp seeds walnuts perilla	*alkalinizing protein sources:* high alpha whey protein isolate powder hemp protein powder pea and soy protein powders
	omega-6 essential fatty acids: borage oil evening primrose oil black currant seed oil	

Fish Oils	Vegetable Oils	Protein
	omega-7 fatty acids: macadamia nuts sea buckthorn berries	
	omega-9 fatty acids: extra virgin olive oil macadamia nut oil	

Bright Yellow Color-Coded Foods

Two or three times a week, to sharpen your memory, rejuvenate brain cells, and ignite healthy bone-building, consume the egg yolks of organic, free-range, vegetable-fed chickens, as well as yellow or orange marigold flower petals in your salads.

Nightshade Vegetables

Many aging conditions cause pain and, surprisingly so, your diet affects pain intensity. Nightshade vegetables are an example.

Phytonutrients in some groups of foods, such as the nightshades, can actually worsen muscle and joint pain in a small portion of the population. Bell peppers, eggplant, potatoes, and tomatoes are members of the nightshade or Solanaceae family. For 95 percent of the population, these foods do not cause a problem. It has also been noted that aged cheese contains tyramines, which elevate monoamine oxidase, reduce the "energizing" hormone dopamine and the "feel good" hormone serotonin, and also cause pain in some people prone to osteoarthritis, who should avoid these foods.

Automatic Sprouter

Daikon sprouts, sunflower sprouts, broccoli sprouts, and pea sprouts are nutrient powerhouses full of ready-to-use phytonutrients. Sprouting seeds provides a great opportunity for you and your children to grow your own food. It is simple to sprout seeds, legumes, or grains indoors, 12 months of the year, even in limited space.

Use organic seeds or grains that have not been pretreated for agricultural purposes. Sprouts are partially predigested and therefore easy to digest. Live enzymes readily available in sprouts add to the stomach's digestive enzymes. Sprouts are extremely nutritious, and an inexpensive way to raise your own organic foods and reduce food costs. Children love to grow live food as sprouts. Today, you can purchase automatic sprouters that operate without the use of soil, have no mold, do not require watering, and are hassle free! See the Product Resources section for a supplier of a five star-rated sprouter.

Medicinal Mushrooms

Medicinal mushrooms contain ancient phytonutrients called polysaccharides, lectins, and terpenoids, which have powerful immune-potentiating effects. The most familiar medicinal mushrooms are cordyceps, maitake, reishi, and shiitake. Mushroom polysaccharides have remarkable anti-tumor activity: Beta-glucan from maitake mushrooms, for example, induces apoptosis (death) in prostate cancer cells.

Fresh Vegetable Juice

Daily, have a glass of vegetable juice to add colorful phytonutrients to your diet.

My favorite vegetable juice recipe, taught to me by my grandma Nana Marie, is:

Grandma Nana Marie's Vegetable Juice Recipe

- 2 medium carrots
- 6 stems each: watercress, cilantro, parsley
- ½ a small red beet
- 1 small red tomato
- 1 tbsp of fresh chopped ginger
- juice of ½ a small lemon
- 1 stalk of celery with leaves
- dash of cayenne or curry or turmeric
- ½ yellow or orange pepper
- 1 clove of garlic (optional)

A Note on Coffee

The optimum amount of organic coffee I recommend is 2 cups per day. Black, organic coffee is alkaline-forming, but once you add a natural or synthetic sweetener the coffee becomes acidic. Caffeine-sensitive people (I am one), who get a severe buzz and jitters on ½ cup of coffee, should avoid it.

Dr. Robert Heaney, of Creighton University, a world authority on bones and osteoporosis, reported in the journal *Food and Chemical Toxicology* in 2002 that there is no evidence of a detrimental effect on calcium absorption, bone health, or osteoporosis as long as an individual meets daily calcium requirements. Most population studies have found no relationship between coffee, tea, and osteoporosis and although they do increase calcium excretion, it is extremely minor.

Danish researchers reported in the *American Journal of Clinical Nutrition* in 2001 that people with an existing heart, stroke, or artery-blockage problem may want to avoid coffee. Two substances in coffee, caffestol and kahweol, appear to be the culprits that can significantly increase cholesterol and homocysteine levels in the bloodstream of some people, leading to an increased risk of stroke, heart disease, and diabetes. If you must consume caffeine, I would recommend black, white, and green tea, which contain significant amounts of bone-building phytonutrients. Scientists at Tufts University have found that a cup of black, white, or matcha green tea has more antioxidant capabilities than a cup of broccoli, carrots, spinach, or strawberries.

Matcha green tea and black tea appear to boost immune functions, help fight cancer, prevent heart disease, and accelerate healthy bone-building. That is a lot of power in a cup of tea. You will feel more relaxed and, hopefully, have a little more peace of mind.

Berry Phytonutrients Rejuvenate Your Brain and Bones

Can you repair and restore the brain's broken and dysfunctional circuits and cell signaling or communication pathways in your bones once some of these functions have been lost? The answer is a resounding *yes!*

In 1999 and in a 2003 follow-up study, Dr. James A. Joseph and researchers from Tufts University found that age-related brain degeneration could be delayed in young animals if they were supplemented with extracts of spinach and strawberries. This was a complete surprise because only strong experimental drugs were thought to be effective in treating brain damage.

Dr. Joseph next experimented with blackberries and blueberries. He chose rats—equivalent in age to 70-year-old humans—with age-related brain deficits that had diminished memory, an impaired sense of balance, and motor-control decline. For eight weeks he fed the rats a regular control diet containing 1–2 percent of calories from either extracts of fresh blueberries, strawberries, or spinach mixed with their regular food.

The totally unthinkable happened. The rats that were fed the strawberries, spinach, or blueberries dramatically reversed their mental deficits, such as stroke and Alzheimer's. Their brains and bones were operating and functioning at much younger levels—back to 40 years of age from 70—in relation to humans! Dr. Joseph was amazed by the results. He had rejuvenated old brains—yes!—with a ½ cup of berries. This is highly significant. You can reverse the telltale signs of brain aging and the insensitivity of receptors in bone and brain cells, and restore eroded integrity of both circuitries to reverse dementia, short-term memory loss, the early stages of Alzheimer's disease, and the degenerative decline in bone-building function. During berry season eat 1 cup of various berries daily. In the off-season you can eat 1 cup of frozen berries.

Eat Tan, Not White, Carbohydrates

Tan foods are important sources of nutrients that are in short supply in our diet, including dietary fiber, trace minerals, phytoestrogens, phytosterols, lignans, and polysaccharides with impressive anti-cancer potential.

White potatoes without their skins (french fries) clearly lack colorful phytonutrients and increase free radicals and damage to bone cells. Dr. Christina Lasheras reported in the *Journal of the American Dietetic Association* in 2003 that tan color-coded whole rice and pasta were not associated with the increases in oxidative damage to cells that occur with french fries. She recommends replacing white potatoes in your diet with whole-grain rice, oven-roasted sweet potato, or yams complete with their skins on. I like to keep baked yams, sweet potatoes, and purple potatoes in the refrigerator and eat them as healthy snacks, skin and all.

The Ancient Green Color Code Is a Powerhouse

Cruciferous (Brassica) vegetables, garlic, and onions release their sulfur compounds and pungent flavor when they are cut up, crushed, or mashed. They protect DNA from damage and stimulate apoptosis (cell death) in colon, breast, and prostate cancer cells. The chlorophyll-intense, ancient green color code is anti-carcinogenic, anti-bacterial, anti-viral, and anti-microbial.

A British research team led by Paul Thornalley, Ph.D., of the University of Essex, discovered a remarkably significant anti-aging property of indols and isothiocyanates in green foods. They inhibit enzymes that promote glycation and formation of advanced glycation end-products (AGEs), which cause proteins to stick together like Velcro. These gooey, sticky proteins cross-link, lose their elasticity, and cause wrinkles in your facial skin. The indols and isothiocyanates have the ability to reverse the wrinkles on your skin and face.

Thiosulfonate and sulphoraphane in green foods, according to Paul Talaly, M.D., of Johns Hopkins University, are powerful inducers of protective enzymes known as Phase 1 and Phase 2 detoxifying enzymes in your liver; they turn toxins into water-soluble, biotransformed, nontoxic substances.

Egg Yolks and Marigolds

The xanthophyll family of bright yellow carotenoids have unusual names like astaxanthin, canthaxanthin, lutein, and zeaxanthin. These carotenes are fat-soluble (lipophilic) and, unlike all other carotenes, they do not convert to vitamin A but remain in the fatty lipid bilayer of cells, protecting the integrity of their membranes from internal or external assaults.

Egg yolks are the only nutrient-dense, bioavailable source of lutein, zeaxanthin, and astaxanthin, which are scavengers of singlet oxygen free radicals. The lutein, zeaxanthin, and astaxanthin from organic, free-range chicken egg yolks is 300 percent more bioavailable than the supplement forms. They are fully reactive and scientific evidence shows that they can easily break down by exposure to high heat or air. Therefore, only soft-boil, hard-boil, or poach eggs so their yolks are left slightly soft. Overcooking denatures and coagulates the protein in eggs, which makes it hard for you to absorb the beneficial protein. Do not scramble eggs or make omelettes that break the yolk and destroy the xanthophyll carotenoids. The high heat of a frying pan is destructive for sensitive xanthophylls and frying causes dangerous cholesterol oxides. Eggs have been redeemed and exonerated by both the American and Canadian Heart Associations. They are back to being a healthy choice. The xanthophyll antioxidants protect the eyes and skin from aberrant, free radical, oxidative stress and sun damage.

The Power of Color-Coded Carotenoids

Six hundred different carotenes (polyphenols in produce with the orange and red color codes) or carotenoids, with a wide variety of names, have been identified. The four most known carotenes are designated by Greek prefixes such as alpha-, beta-, delta-, and gamma-carotene. All four carotenes are precursors of vitamin A.

Today, research scientists believe the most important benefits of lipophilic (fat-soluble) carotenoids are their powerful antioxidant capacity. They have an intense affinity to enter the lipid bilayer membrane (layers of fat, then water, then fat), which covers all cells, and successfully trap free radicals that are generated within the cell or that try to gain entry from outside. Recently, the carotenoids have been found to stabilize cell-to-cell communication and signaling transduction pathways, which is the basis for many of their anti-cancer, anti-inflammatory, immune-strengthening, and enhanced bone-building effects. As antioxidants they minimize random free radical destructive reactions in bone cells.

Various colored members of the carotenoid family have preferences for protecting specific cellular membranes, membrane receptors, and particular cellular signaling pathways:

- Lycopene (from tomatoes, red raspberries, pink grapefruit, beets, black bing cherries, dark red grapes, and red Swiss chard) protects the prostate gland, brain neurons, and bone micro-architecture.

- Astaxanthin, lutein, and zeaxanthin (from egg yolks and marigolds) protect the eyes from macular degeneration, cataracts, the effects of ultraviolet radiation, and endogenous free radical formation.

- Canthaxanthin and astaxanthin (from egg yolks and marigolds), and lycopene (from red carotenoid foods) are most protective of the skin against radiation from ultraviolet A (UVA) and ultraviolet B (UVB) sunrays and sunburn.

- Curcumin (*Curcuma longa*), the active ingredient in the spice turmeric (which gives curry its flavor and golden color), is unquestionably related to beta-carotene and reduces systemic inflammation and protects against cancer in general.

- Alpha-, beta-, delta-, and gamma-carotene (from carrots, tomatoes, yams, squash, and red lettuce) protect all cells (like bone cells) from oxidative damage and free radical attacks, playing a crucial role in the early prevention of atherosclerosis, rheumatoid arthritis, and osteoporosis.

The xanthophyll family of carotenes, or carotenoids, can be taken as supplements, especially if you are going to expose your eyes or skin to sunlight. Natural mixed carotenoids extracted from sea vegetables, such as *Spirulina pacifica* and *Daniella salina*, are available in softgels from 5,000–10,000 IU. Lutein and zeaxanthin are available in softgels extracted from yellow and orange marigolds in strengths from 2–6 mg. Lycopene, extracted from red tomatoes, is available in softgels from 2–15 mg. Astaxanthin, canthaxanthin, beta-cryptoxanthin, or phytofluene are available (generally only astaxanthin is available) in softgels at 2–4 mg. I highly suggest you supplement with astaxanthin if you plan to expose your skin to sunrays for an extended period of time.

Essential Fatty Acids: Ancient, Beneficial Phytonutrients for Cellular Membranes

Fatty acids make up the lipid bilayer of all cellular membranes, including those in living bone tissue. Oxidative free radical damage to these critical lipids (fats) causes both a faulty and a dramatic downgrade in cell-to-cell communication and cellular absorption potentials. These specialized fats (from small fish like anchovies, herring, mackerel, and sardines from clean, cold waters off the coast of South America) are called eicosapentaenoic acid (EPA) and "bone-building" docosahexaenoic acid (DHA). These beneficial and ancient fats are called long-chain omega-3 essential fatty acids. Your body cannot make them.

Researchers once believed we could convert the short-chain omega-3 essential fatty acids from flaxseed oil to the long-chain form we need, but Dr. Bruce Holub, Ph.D., University of Guelph, in Ontario, Canada, discovered that humans convert only 5–20 percent of flax oil to long-chain omega-3s and we need to "leapfrog" over flaxseed oil and use fish oils daily.

Moving at close to 150 mph and zigzagging with precision, hormones, growth hormones, minerals, trace minerals, and phytonutrients rely on specific receptor sites embedded deep in the lipid bilayer of membranes to relay messages and for uptake. Any distortion of the cellular membrane microenvironment or free radical assaults leads to faulty gene expressions and the receptor sites will be unavailable to transmit, absorb, or transport messages across cell membranes.

Long-chain omega-3 essential fatty acid supplements from fish oils are particularly effective in stabilizing cell membranes and effectively reduce the risk of cardiovascular disease, depression, memory loss, and osteoporosis in both men and women. They also downgrade learning disabilities ADD and ADHD. The EPA and DHA fats in fish oils accelerate healthy bone-building.

Prescriptions for Specific Omega-3, -6, -7, and -9 Supplements

Trying to maintain healthy bone strength, tall structure, good posture, and fluid biomechanical movement without fish oils rich in the biologically active long-chain omega-3 essential fatty acids EPA and DHA is like trying to build the sturdiest brick house in town with weak, crumbly bricks. You may have the best architect, the best contractor, and the best location, but if you do not have strong bricks, your dream house will not be built properly and the foundation will be weak and prone to crumble.

The EPA fraction of fish oils has been shown to boost good moods, alleviate depression, indecisiveness, and learning disabilities while raising the brain's production of two "good-mood" brain messengers serotonin and dopamine. The DHA fraction of fish oils has been well researched to build stronger structural scaffolding in the brain to boost the production of more brain cells and enhance the brain's ability to significantly remember, learn, and communicate. Furthermore, "bone-smart" DHA also builds stronger structural scaffolding in the micro-architecture of our 206 bones.

What Your Bones Love

In the 1990s, positive research found that fish oil was a "new" miracle cure for osteoarthritis and osteoporosis. Studies also proved that fish oil reduces pain significantly by inhibiting pro-inflammatory chemicals your body makes like cyclooxygenase (COX-2) and prostaglandin E2 (PGE2). At high levels, PGE2 aggravates aching joints and damages healthy osteoblast (bone-building) cells.

Low levels of PGE2, according to Carolyn DeMarco, M.D., increases the production of insulin-like growth factors, a "master" growth stimulator for bone, cartilage, and muscle tissue.

Dr. Bruce Wadkins, of Purdue University, reported in the 2001 edition of *Experimental Biology and Medicine* that there are "Consistent and reproducible beneficial effects of long-chain omega-3 fats (fish oil) on bone metabolism and bone joint diseases."

Quite amazingly so, two other super-critical healthy fats—omega-7 fats from macadamia nut and oil—and omega-9 fats from olive oil or macadamia nut oil reduce systemic inflammation and accelerate bone growth, bone density, and bone strength.

What Fish Oil Supplement Is Best for Bone Growth?

My recommendation is that you supplement daily with enteric-coated softgels of fish oil for better absorption or a liquid fish oil that combines omega-3, -6, -7, and -9 essential fats based on the research of Dr. Alan C. Logan, a faculty member of Harvard Medical School's Mind-Body Institute. Dr. Logan has developed a breakthrough solution for us to receive all our essential fats and to successfully build bone tissue by developing an omega-3 product made of premium omega-3, omega-6, omega-7, and omega-9 sources.

Three enteric-coated softgels taken once a day with any meal contain:

- omega-3 EPA, 324 mg
- omega-3 DHA, 216 mg

- omega-6 GLA, 180 mg
- omega-7, 276 mg
- omega-9, 588 mg

Note 1: Many fish oil supplements are now available in a good-tasting, naturally flavored liquid format for children, seniors, or those who prefer a liquid over a softgel.

Note 2: Krill (*Euphausia superba*) are very small Antarctic shrimp-like zooplankton that are another popular source of EPA and DHA essential fats. However, the magazine *Nature*, in November 2004, published research that krill in the Antarctic have been overharvested, decreasing their volume by 70 percent and leaving inadequate amounts for whales. Therefore, I do not recommend that you use krill oil supplements.

Where to find your best fats

Type of Fat	Daily Source
lignans and short-chain omega-3 fats	2 tbsps of both flax and sesame seeds ground in a coffee grinder and added to your breakfast protein shake
biologically active long-chain omega-3 fats	three softgels daily, of enteric-coated fish oils, high in "mood-smart" EPA and "bone-smart" DHA, one at breakfast, lunch, and supper
biologically active omega-6 fats as the important gamma-linolenic acid (GLA)	1,200 mg of borage oil contained in three fish oil softgels or ½ tsp of borage oil or ¾ tsp of black currant seed oil or 1,000 mg of evening primrose oil taken once a day with a meal
omega-7 fats	six to 10 macadamia nuts (or ⅛ tsp sea buckthorn oil) or macadamia oil
omega-9 fats	2 tbsps of organic extra virgin olive oil on your salads or vegetables and use stable macadamia nut oil for cooking

Note: For great taste and cooking or baking, the newest healthy oil is macadamia nut oil. The vitamin E content of macadamia nut oil is four times that of olive oil, and it is extremely heat stable because of its high level of monounsaturated fatty acids.

> Color-coded fruits, vegetables, salads, sprouts, culinary herbs, and spices are abundant year-round. Autumn and winter fruits and vegetables exposed to frost are sweeter and contain higher levels of all phytonutrients.

All foods from these six ancient color-coded categories are especially powerful antioxidants that are at the forefront against free radicals generated from air pollution, tobacco smoke, exercise, natural biochemical processes, industrial chemicals, and psychological stress. These colorful phytonutrients are anti-inflammatory, anti-carcinogenic, protect the brain and central nervous system, and are photoprotective of the sun's harmful ultraviolet rays on your skin in a weakening ozone layer.

Culinary Herbs and Spices

Culinary herbs and spices are flavorful phytonutrients that dramatically improve a sluggish metabolism and help to digest foods. Examples are curries, garlic, cinnamon, ginger, cayenne, nutmeg, turmeric, basil, oregano, thyme, sage, mint, bay leaf, mint, peppermint, marjoram, rosemary, and tarragon. Do not keep herbs and spices in your kitchen for too long as dried herbs and spices lose their flavor and antioxidant properties within 60 days.

The antioxidant capacity of 15 culinary herbs out of a rating of 100, the ideal antioxidant capacity	
1. Southwest oregano	92.18
2. Italian oregano	71.64
3. Greek oregano	64.71
4. Sweet bay leaf	31.70
5. Dill	29.12
6. Winter savory	26.34
7. Vietnamese coriander	22.90
8. Orange mint	19.80
9. Garden thyme	19.49
10. Ginkgo biloba	19.18
11. Rosemary	19.15
12. Lemon verbena	17.88
13. Sweet basil	14.27
14. Garden sage	12.28
15. Parsley	11.03

Use these culinary herbs liberally in your meal planning. Use fresh herbs, such as oregano, rosemary, dill, coriander, parsley, sweet basil, mint, and thyme, in your salads. Use nonirradiated, organic dry herbs, such as oregano, dill, sage, mint, pineapple sage, chives, thyme, and basil on your vegetables. Add fresh herbs to all your cooked dishes to add unique flavors, medicinal healing and aroma, and to aid digestion. Once hooked on indispensable herbs, you will want a backyard herbal garden, or a large pot or window box garden of fresh herbs. I do all three—*bon appétit!*

Spices

Today, spices remain as important to daily well-being as they did to all the early explorers, navigators, and trade merchants who plied the high seas in the wealthy trade of exotic culinary spices. Do you use spices? Perhaps you use them more than you know: Garlic and black pepper are a standard in most ethnic cultures' fine foods; cardamom, cinnamon, cloves, and black pepper flavor chai tea; ginger, nutmeg, cinnamon, and cloves are ingredients in pumpkin pie; ginger is instrumental in Thai cuisine; turmeric, cumin, cloves, cinnamon, fenugreek, garlic, and chilies are used in curry; cardamom, allspice, and cinnamon are elements in apple pie; cloves are used in deodorant; eggnog contains nutmeg; and black pepper, cumin, chilies, and garlic are found in Mexican sauces.

Spices may be the most potent disease fighters available and can make your food choices delicious. Experiment with spices daily as their disease-fighting compounds remain intact even when they are heated and used in cooking.

- **Black pepper** stimulates hydrochloric acid secretion in the stomach to improve digestion and has potent antibacterial properties.

- **Cardamom** is actually an aromatic herb that has anti-viral, anti-bacterial, anti-fungal, anti-Candida capacities.

- **Cinnamon,** in a placebo-controlled study, inhibited free radicals by 88 percent. Cinnamon normalizes blood sugar levels—½ tsp a day reduces blood glucose levels in diabetics by 40 percent. Cinnamon can lower the glycemic load of any meal or breakfast protein power drink. (The glycemic load is determined by calculating the amount of carbohydrate in a particular food and its impact on blood glucose levels and insulin levels.)

- **Fenugreek** seeds are used extensively in Ayurvedic medicine to treat both diabetes and obesity. Fenugreek stabilizes high blood sugar levels and has anti-microbial and anti-cancer properties.

- **Ginger** has amazingly effective anti-inflammatory capabilities. It contains a polyphenol called zingibain, which has almost 1,000 percent more protein-digesting power than the commonly used digestive enzymes in papaya, and is an effective and widely used treatment for both rheumatoid arthritis and an upset stomach.

- **Turmeric** is the famous, brilliant golden-yellow color in curry powder and the darling of medical researchers globally. It has been used for centuries in Chinese and Ayurvedic medicine to treat gastrointestinal and inflammatory ailments. Turmeric and ginger work synergistically and are a much safer anti-inflammatory alternative than aspirin and ibuprofen (standard nonsteroidal anti-inflammatory drugs, or NSAIDs). Turmeric, especially its curcumin polyphenol component, possesses unbelievable capabilities in the prevention and treatment of cancer as it arrests the growth of cancer cells at the G2 stage of their cell division.

Three Herbs in Capsules That You Need in Your Medicine Cabinet

These medicinal herbs as supplements are found in all natural food stores.

- **Butterbur** is a perennial herb with a phytonutrient called *petasin,* which quells muscle spasms in vascular walls and traditionally is used to manage bronchial asthma and hay fever (allergic rhinitis). Research published in the journal *Neurology* in December 2004 proved that 22 mg of petasin reduced migraine headaches by 61 percent.

- **Rhodiola** rosea has been clinically proven to help balance the stress-response system, reducing anxiety and overreactivity, enabling people to remain calmer and cope better whether they have normal or overactive stress-response systems.

- **Vinpocetine** is derived from the periwinkle plant (Vinca minor), which is used successfully in various forms of dementia, acute stroke, and urinary inconsistency or incontinence.

PART 3:
MARKETING FADS—BUYER BEWARE

Lun Lun and Yang Yang have needs that are met each day with diverse color-coded, "cell-friendly" vegetables and fruits. They each eat an all-vegetarian diet—84 lbs a day. Lun Lun and Yang Yang are a pair of star-attraction pandas at the Atlanta, Georgia, Zoo. We have some budgetary breathing room because we require only 2 lbs of fresh, color-coded, "cell-friendly" fruits, vegetables, salads, "green drinks," herbs, and spices a day. We should consume three servings (a serving is 1 cup) of fruits or berries and six to eight servings (a serving is 1 cup) of colorful vegetables and salads daily.

Nutritional Fads: Wolves in Sheep's Clothing

A walk down any grocery aisle in North America is an instant study in nutritional fads: low carbs, low sodium, low sugar, and low cholesterol, but none as lucrative and enduring as low fat.

According to ProductScan Online, in 2005, 12.8 percent of all new food products were emblazoned with a low-fat or fat-free label. In 1998, at the height of the low-fat phenomenon, 51 percent of all consumers said they were "very" or "extremely" concerned about reducing fat in their diet. In 2005, according to Health Focus International, a marketing research firm that specializes in health trends, only 31 percent were worried about reducing fats in their diet.

The food industry is likely to be busy reformulating and marketing processed food products to incorporate the latest nutritional thinking about fats. Yes, there are good and bad fats. The good include extra virgin olive oil (an omega-9 fat); macadamia nuts or sea buckthorn oil (an omega-7 fat); borage, evening primrose, or black currant seed oil (an omega-6 fat); "mood-smart" EPA and "bone-smart" DHA-rich fats from fish oils like anchovies, sardines, and mackerel (long-chain omega-3 fats) and extra virgin coconut oil to use as butter. The bad are trans fats, which are found in partially hydrogenated oil, acrylamides found in fried starchy foods like french fries, and saturated fats found in animal fats.

The shift toward a greater acceptance of dietary fat, initially prompted by the Atkins diet, has been underway for several years.

Hoping to capitalize on consumers' desires for healthier fats, some commercial food companies are starting to change the way they produce and market processed products. In the last few years, most food manufacturers have mounted major efforts to take out trans fat, which scientists and nutritionists consider to be the worst kind of fat. They are replacing them with potentially rancid substitutes like soybean oil, canola oil, and palm oil.

You must be very careful because the marketing muscle and strategies employed by some food processors sound nutritionally attractive, but they still remove ancient, critical, "cell-friendly" components and colorful phytonutrients. Marketing and packaging pizzazz is no substitute for genuine, healthful foods.

The Biotech Gap between Lab and Table Widens

In 1977 the North American public saw its first television commercial for water. Orson Wells talked about a place in the south of France where "there is a spring, and its name is Perrier," and North American sales rose by more than 3,000 percent from 1976 to 1979.

The Beverage Marketing Corp., the water industry's main research group, says that North Americans spent more than $10 billion U.S. on bottled water in 2005.

The forests of France, the hills of Maine, and the glaciers in the Canadian Rockies quickly evolved into "Icelandic glaciers" and "Pacific aquifers." Yet, 40 percent of bottled waters are made from just municipal tap water; marketers tout arcane methods of distillation and filtration and add an assortment of minerals to get that exact "watery" taste.

An increasing number of health and environmental groups are challenging the nutritional claims and also the harmlessness of the bottled-water business—and so should you!

The High-Performance Superdrink—Yes!—Water

Crystal-clean water is one of the sweetest things imaginable. You should drink a minimum of six 8 oz glasses of water a day, and more if the weather is hot, if you perspire more, or if you exercise for more than 30 minutes. Often we misinterpret thirst signals as hunger signs and we eat when we really should be drinking water. Our skin is 80 percent water, our brain is 74 percent, and even our solid bones are 22 percent water.

Do not wait to drink your water quota for the day all at once. Your body's need for water is constant. Prehydrate by drinking water every two hours. Do what I do—I carry an enclosed container with a straw in it and leave it on my desk as I work and take it in my vehicle. Only oxygen is more essential to sustaining life. You can live for 35 to 50 days without food, but only three to five days without water.

Your household water is probably chlorinated and fluorinated by your municipality. The chlorine and fluoride that are added to kill bacteria, which means they kill all bacteria, even the beneficial bacteria in your intestines, can cause digestive and absorption problems.

To protect your family, I strongly recommend that you install one of the several available household water filters in your home or purchase bottled water. The best way to maintain the quality of your drinking water is to invest in a home water-treatment system. Tap water costs less than .01 cents per gallon, bottled water costs approximately $1.50 per gallon, reverse osmosis systems 20 cents per gallon, acid alkaline machines 30 cents per gallon, and steam distillation 25 cents per gallon. When it is all said and done, the choice is between reverse osmosis and distillation water units. In either case, ensure that your system has an ultraviolet light attached to the water line that kills all bacteria and viruses. Do not be discouraged by the cost of a water-treatment unit, which may run from $250 to $2,000. They may seem expensive, but no more so than other major appliances like refrigerators, stoves, washers, and dryers. Don't hesitate to purchase a proper water-treatment system.

Gray Hair and Weak Bones are Linked

The graying of our hair can tell us plenty about what is going on inside our bones. A study published in 2005 in the *Journal of Clinical Endocrinology and Metabolism*, linked premature graying of hair to the thinning of our bones. People under the age of 45 who are starting to show signs of gray hair would be wise to use a food-based, bone-building supplement to ignite healthy bone-building and prevent any further deterioration of bone strength—and hopefully reverse the premature graying of their hair.

CHAPTER 7

Developing an Alkaline Bone-Building Diet

THE ALKALINE PUZZLE

Your body is a very complicated and miraculous chemical processing plant with 100 trillion cells involved in some 8 trillion chemical reactions each second. An alkaline environment is necessary for optimal health and ideal biochemical functioning. As you study the easy-to-use pH chart in this chapter (page 193), note that most of the favorite processed fast foods, junk foods, and soft drinks are acid forming. Alkaline balance is very important for bone health. We evolved in an alkaline ocean environment and even today the body's internal environment remains alkaline, with a pH just above 7. Our 206 bones and 143 joints' enzymatic, immunological, and repair mechanisms all function at their best in an alkaline environment that maintains biochemical balance called homeostasis.

Homeostasis is the internal dialogue going on in all 100 trillion cells, a give-and-take relationship coupling acidic and alkaline partners in the rhythmic dance of life. Many of the factors known to increase acidity also cause systemic inflammation, which has been shown to accelerate aging. Acidity and excessive inflammation apparently go hand in hand—alkalinity and reduced inflammation also go hand in hand. The best way to decrease the production of silent inflammation-promoting chemicals called cytokines and leukotrienes is maintaining an alkaline edge by eating brightly colored produce.

While an internal alkaline balance is optimal, our biochemical functioning, the processes of living, and the metabolism of food produce a great deal of acid. For example, when we exercise or move, we produce lactic acid. At the same time, we will also produce carbonic acid, which further increases acidity and eventually breaks down to carbon dioxide and water.

When we eat, we generate acids. For example, sulfuric acid can be produced from the metabolism of sulfur-containing amino acids when we eat animal protein, and when we consume phosphoric acid in food, especially pop or spritzers. Furthermore, immune responses such as allergies and hypersensitivity, and even stress, anxiety, and sleeplessness generate substantial amounts of acidic by-products.

To regain the life-supporting alkaline state, metabolic acids from all sources must be buffered or neutralized with salts of alkaline minerals. For example, potassium citrate and potassium malate are salts of organic anions commonly found in vegetables and fruits. These organic anions, when metabolized, can accept hydrogen ions and thus reduce and neutralize the acid load and create an alkaline balance.

Bone contributes to the maintenance of our all-important alkaline/acid balance by buffering a portion of the acid generated from the metabolism of food. Bone contains a large reservoir of potentially mobilizable alkaline salts of calcium, sodium, magnesium, and potassium. When our internal pH turns acidic, these minerals are mobilized from bone to neutralize excess acidity. Prolonged and repeated utilization of alkaline minerals for acid neutralization can deplete bone and contribute to osteoporosis and a loss of fluid mobility. Thus, those with a more acidifying chemistry waste mineral reserves in mandatory pH balancing.

While the link between an acid pH and osteoporosis has been known for some time, the topic has been the subject of serious investigation only recently.

THE EVER-PRESENT ACID CULPRITS

The human body is composed of 68 percent water. The cells in the body are 90 percent water. The body fluids of healthy people are slightly alkaline while the same fluids of those who are sick range from slightly to extremely acidic. The degree of acidity significantly affects the body's ability to prevent and/or reverse illness and disease, including such degenerative diseases as cancer, diabetes, heart disease, and osteoporosis. In my first book *The Power of Superfoods*, I highly recommend that in order to avoid disease and premature aging, the body should remain in a slightly alkaline condition.

The standard North American diet consists of a lot of processed fast foods that are low in protein, but high in fat, salt, sugar, high-fructose corn sweeteners, artificial sweeteners, and white carbohydrates, which contribute to an overly acidic body. Another source of acid is cola soft drinks, which have an acidic range around 2.5 pH. It takes an incredible amount of "good" water to counteract the effects of one cola. In other words, you may have to drink nearly 32 glasses of 7.0 pH water to eliminate the bad effects of one glass of pop. In addition to pop, stress, meat, sweetened coffee, sugar sweeteners, sugar substitutes, overexercising, lack of sleep, acute stress, and smoking all contribute to raising the acid levels in one's body, thereby contributing to serious health problems.

Many people erroneously think that kidney stones are caused by excessive calcium. The real culprit may be the high level of phosphoric acid in the diet, which is the primary ingredient in soft drinks. The body uses calcium leached from bones to convert poisonous liquid phosphoric acid into the more stable solid phosphate form. Phosphates can form into calcified kidney stones.

It is important to understand that changing the body's pH does not cure disease; however, it allows the body to heal itself by ridding it of toxins and adding the minerals that are so important to maintaining good health. Leon Root, M.D., in *Beautiful Bones without Hormones*, states, "Even a small drop in the body's pH can cause a dramatic increase in bone loss."

MONITORING YOUR MORNING ACID-ALKALINE BALANCE

The first step in establishing a health-promoting alkaline diet is to assess your current pH. A good measure of average body pH is easily obtained by assessing the pH of your first morning urine or saliva before you drink any liquid or brush your teeth.

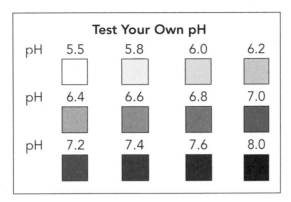

Figure 7.1: Test Your Own pH

1. Obtain a packet of pH hydrion test paper. This test tape measures acid-alkaline states and should be marked into one-half point divisions ranging at least from 5.5 to 8.0. See Product Resources for a source.

2. First thing in the morning, just before your first urination, open the test tape packet and cut off 2 or 3 inches of the paper tape. Now wet the test tape with urine, or you can use your saliva. Do not put the pH test paper in your mouth, but simply put your saliva onto a saucer and dip the pH paper into it.

3. As the tape is moistened with urine or saliva, it will take on a color. The color relates to an acid or alkaline state and ranges from yellow to dark blue. Match the color of your test strip with the color chart on the back of the test tape packet.

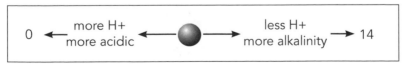

Figure 7.2: Acid and Alkalinity

Day	pH Reading	30-Day pH Test Journal	Day	pH Reading
1			16	
2			17	
3			18	
4		An ideal range	19	
5		for first morning	20	
6		urine pH should be	21	
7		between 6.8 and 7.4	22	
8			23	
9		An ideal first	24	
10		morning saliva pH	25	
11		should be between	26	
12		6.6 and 6.8	27	
13			28	
14			29	
15			30	

4. Jot down the number that corresponds to the color your tape has taken on. Any number below 7 means that your urine or saliva is on the acidic side. The lower the number, the more acid the condition. For example, a number of 6.0 indicates considerable acidity while 6.8 indicates much less. A number of 7 indicates the neutral state, neither acid or alkaline.

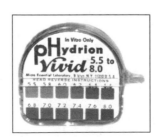

Figure 7.3: pH Paper

Ideally the first morning urine pH should be between a pH of 6.8 and 7.4, or the first morning saliva between 6.6 and 6.8. When the first morning urine is neutral or just slightly acidic, this indicates that the overall cellular pH is appropriately alkaline.

5. If your readings fall below 6.6, you should begin changes aimed at alkalinizing your diet. Below are listed simple dietary modifications that will help alkalinize your diet. In the beginning, because of the acid-forming tendency of the standard North American diet, most people will have low pH readings. On the other hand, there will be an occasional person whose pH readings are always highly alkaline (greater than 7.5). Generally, these people are not consuming sufficient daily protein in their diet. A knowledgeable health professional can provide more information for you.

Your pH Level May Dictate Your Moods and Intelligence

Your pH levels can have an impact on your mental state. Prayer, quiet meditation, Qigong, Tai Chi, reflexology, massage therapy, shiatsu, acupuncture, breathing exercises, therapeutic touch, calming music, hatha yoga, walking in nature, deeply appreciating nature, reaching out to others with love and sincere compassion—all these activities help to promote a calm, alkaline body by raising your "tending and befriending" hormone oxytocin and reducing acidifying cortisol.

Researchers have found that people who keep a slightly alkaline internal pH tend to be more satisfied and satiated by their diets than those who are eating a more acidifying diet. Furthermore, I recommend that people limit their intake of acidifying foods because they also contain a significant amount of unnecessary calories.

Similarly, your body's pH level may affect your mental abilities. Researchers at the John Radcliffe Hospital in Oxford, England, believe intelligence may be directly linked to pH levels in the brain's cortex. Using a magnetic resonance scanner the team measured the pH in the cortexes of 42 teens. The teens then completed a widely used IQ test. The results showed that those with pH readings of 7 or more had significantly higher IQ levels. This is the first time that intelligence has been linked to a pH biochemical marker in the brain.

ALKALINITY ENHANCES SUPERIOR BONE-BUILDING

Your brain and body's circuitry are extremely sensitive to the slightest change in the pH level of your body's vital fluids. The pH scale runs from 1 to 14: a pH less than 7 is acidic; more than 7 is alkaline. Your body works hard to sustain several pH levels in various body systems. For example, your body wants to maintain an intracellular pH of 6.8 to 7.2 inside your cells. The important extra-cellular pH of your blood is strictly controlled between 7.35 and 7.45 and is slightly alkaline. Your stomach fluid must be acidic, with a pH of 1.5 so it can digest food, but pancreatic fluid is very alkaline with a pH of 8.8.

> Your body, with a great degree of ancient intelligence, maintains a pH balance within very strict parameters, in the same way your body's temperature is to be maintained at 98.6 degrees Fahrenheit.

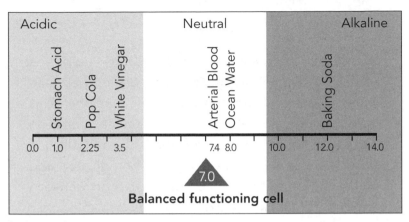

Figure 7.4: Acid-Alkaline Scale

Every day, your body produces organic, acidic by-products such as acetic acid, carbonic acid, fatty acids, lactic acid, and uric acid, which it buffers or neutralizes with organic minerals from the vegetables, salads, herbs, spices, "green drinks," and fruit you eat. When your body's alkaline buffers are not eaten in sufficient daily quantities, toxic, acidic waste accumulates in the cells, causing enormous damage to your overall health. A comprehensive review comparing alkalinizing diets to acidic diets in the *American Journal of Clinical Nutrition* (no. 68, 1998) concludes that alkalinizing diets improve health, nitrogen balance, bone density, and human growth hormone (HGH) concentrations. Acidic diets cause acidosis (low oxygen levels), bone loss (osteoporosis), and muscle mass loss. Acidosis appears to allow pathogens and cancer cells to proliferate, whereas an alkaline pH (high oxygen levels) discourages cancer cell promotion.

Acid-forming foods keep your central nervous system in a hypervigilant and stressful state. This causes your adrenal glands to work overtime, which eventually depletes adrenal reserves and gives you that

---

Alkaline Water

Besides an alkalinizing diet, another interesting option to help create an alkaline pH is by drinking alkaline water, made with an alkaline water machine. This small compact device contains an electrical ionization system to split the water into its acidic and alkaline portions. The water's alkalinity can be adjusted and you can increase the level gradually to a pH between 9.5 and 10. Drink the alkaline water. Use the acidic water for washing your acid-loving skin or watering plants, which thrive on acid water. A good-quality alkaline water machine will cost about $500 U.S. and it will last 10 years. See the Product Resources section at the back of the book for a supplier.

"drop-dead fatigue." Alkaline-forming foods promote a healthy state of adrenal function. This pH allows you to feel passionate about life and fully energized.

Measuring the pH of a food as it exists outside of the body is irrelevant. After a food is consumed, digested, and absorbed, the final residue or "ash" is either alkaline, acidic, or neutral depending on the mineral mix in the food. The minerals sulfur, phosphorus, and iron form acid ions once inside the body. These minerals are found primarily in proteins, such as fish, poultry, meat, eggs, dairy, grains, legumes, and most nuts and seeds. These foods are called acid-forming foods. Eating too many of these foods imposes a net acidic overload on the body. The most acid-forming foods are cola soft drinks, animal protein, and alcohol, which are full of phosphoric and carbonic acids. If you consume too many of these foods, your body will work hard to neutralize them with alkaline blood buffers, which then will not be available to neutralize other acidic products your body naturally produces as a by-product of cellular metabolism.

Sodium, potassium, calcium, and magnesium form alkaline reactions once inside the body. These minerals are found primarily in fruits, salads, vegetables, herbs, spices, and "green drinks," and are called alkaline-forming foods.

Note that not all acidic foods increase acidity inside your body. Lemon juice and apple cider vinegar are extremely acidic, with a pH of 3.5, because of their citric acid content. However, in digestion the citric acid breaks apart, and the potassium and magnesium form alkaline ions called potassium or magnesium citrate, which actually increase alkalinity.

THE 75-TO-25 RATIO: AT THE CROSS-ROADS OF YOUR FUTURE HEALTH

You need a daily 75-to-25 percent ratio, so try to consume approximately 75 percent alkaline-forming foods and 25 percent acid-forming foods. Metabolic acidosis (too acidic) or alkalemia (too alkaline) accelerates cellular, biological aging, and prevents peak network neuro-peptide and neurotransmitter communication. Keeping body fluids in acid/alkaline equilibrium is accomplished by: (1) encouraging the neutralizing or buffering systems in the blood like sodium bicarbonate and potassium bicarbonate; (2) regulating the pH action of the lungs; and (3) regulating the pH action of the kidneys, which excrete more or less bicarbonate. The *American Journal of Clinical Nutrition* in 2005 states that a diet high in fruits and vegetables (and "green drinks") reduces net acid production from eating proteins such as meat, and is correlated to higher bone mass and bone mineral density by making more alkaline buffers in your bloodstream like potassium bicarbonate, an "acid sponge."

It is interesting to note that human cells are slightly alkaline and plant cells are slightly acidic. Plant cells leave an alkaline "ash" after being digested. If the human body remains in an acidic state for too long, human cells become acidic like plant cells, facilitating the initiation of cancer cell colonies and osteoporosis.

When you work or exercise hard you create an abundance of volatile liquid acids, so the depth and rate of your breathing automatically increase to remove carbonic acid by separating it into water and CO_2, exhaling CO_2 (carbon dioxide) through the lungs. Then the kidneys kick in by buffering excess acids that are then excreted in the urine with bicarbonates and expelling them.

Respiration—breathing deeply to oxygenate all of your deep tissues and 100 trillion cells—is the primary buffering system in the body. That is why I encourage you to take meaningful pauses daily and to breathe in deeply the revitalizing, alkaline oxygen while removing stale, acidic carbon dioxide. Eating "cell-friendly" foods and deep breathing greatly aid the body's detoxification system and can keep your bones strong and your body cancer free.

In 2003 the journal *Neoplasma* detailed a study in which highly acidifying soft drinks, alcohol, and sweetened coffee proved to be statistically significant risk factors for cancer. Remember, black organic coffee at a maximum of 2 cups per day is alkaline forming. The *American Journal of Clinical Nutrition* presented research demonstrating that alkaline-forming foods build strong bones and prevent risk of fracture and osteoporosis, while an excess of acidifying foods increase bone loss, risk of fracture, and osteoporosis.

Researchers from the University of California demonstrated that potassium alkali salts present in plant foods neutralized the body's acid level and decreased urine calcium excretion (UcaV). They concluded that people eating five servings of vegetables daily could reaccumulate the equivalent of nearly 5 percent of their bone calcium. Previously, the same research team found that "cell-friendly," color-coded plant foods made the body alkaline and protected against hip fracture, and that hip fracture incidence correlates inversely with the ratio of plant-to-animal food intake—the alkaline/acid balance.

Fruits are classified generally as alkaline due to the presence of citric, malic, and succinic acids, which, after digestion, absorption, and metabolism are converted into bicarbonate and water. Cranberries are an exception. Cranberries are rich sources of phenolic and benzoic acids that do not convert to bicarbonates but are excreted as acids. This is why cranberries are good for urinary infections as the acids literally lift invading bacteria up off the bladder walls where vitamin C from the cranberries can deactivate and destroy the bacteria. The ability of foods to impact the acid-alkaline balance can be measured in your body through the Potential Renal Acid Load (PRAL) test. In 2001 Dr. D.E. Sellameyer reported in the *American Journal of Nutrition* that "A high ratio of dietary animal to vegetable protein increases the rate of bone loss and the risk of fractures." In addition, he says,

"Vegetable foods supply predominantly alkaline (base) precursors. Imbalance between dietary acid and alkaline precursors leads to a chronic net dietary acid load that has adverse consequences on bone health."

DAILY STRESS: A SILENT BONE THIEF

Stress stimulates the "fight-or-flight" response that is a series of lifesaving molecular reactions that protect you from injury or infection. However, chronic stress forces the body to stay on "red alert," sacrificing energy and nutrients targeted for bone-building and redirecting them to a survival mode during acute stressful periods.

In an amazing feedback loop, the adrenal glands kick in to produce cortisol during stress. The more stressful our lifestyle and the poorer our diet, the higher cortisol levels will rise. Cortisol is extremely acidic and corrosive to your bones, muscles, thymus gland, and the hypothalamus (decision-making) part of the brain. Stress increases pro-inflammatory signaling factors called eicosanoids, which disrupt and garble bone-building signals and communication. The *American Journal of Physiological Renal Physiology* proved that stress, accompanied by elevated cortisol, slowed bone-building and dramatically increased bone-breakdown functions.

An alkaline diet blunts the quantitative damage and the cell-to-cell communication havoc that elevated cortisol can have on healthy bone metabolism.

THE EQUILIBRIUM THEORY: ACID/ALKALINE HOMEOSTASIS

The acid-alkaline balance could be called the equilibrium theory to make it easy to understand and easy to use as a general principle of health. We may not be able to clarify chemistry or where the exact chemistry takes place, but we have a model of biochemical functions and how they interact. The "feedback loop" between acids consumed that turn "on" production of alkaline salts produces stability and equilibrium in a physiological system, a process called biological homeostasis. Health in any system of cells, especially bone cells, must be in perfect internal balance. Eating more colorful vegetables, salads, berries, melons, fruit, herbs, spices, and "green drinks" is the smartest way to achieve this biological balance. In the January 2006 issue of *The Lancet*, an article, "Eat Your Fruit and Vegetables," reported that six or more servings of fresh fruit and vegetables daily produced 26 percent fewer strokes and heart disease, and a more stable homeostasis, thus reducing osteoporosis.

Your body, with a great degree of ancient intelligence, maintains arterial blood pH balance within very strict parameters between 7.35 and 7.45, in the same way your body's temperature is to be maintained at 98.6 degrees Fahrenheit.

Your body's inner guidance system (biochemical homeostasis) seeks out balance. Indeed, it is astonishing what the body does to try to keep internal, metabolic balance at all costs. When people drink margaritas (acidifying), they instinctively use salt and lime (alkalinizing). When people consume a meal of cooked red

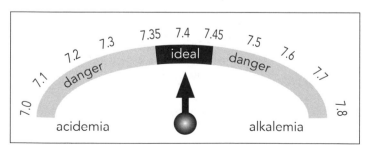

Figure 7.5: Arterial Blood Acid-Base Balance

meat (acidifying), they traditionally like black coffee (alkalinizing) and salt (alkalinizing). What a remarkable body you have—just wonderful!

Your dog will eat grass (alkalinizing) to try to neutralize or buffer the excessive acidity of a high-protein, high-grain diet. Experiment. Mix 1 tsp of an unflavored "green drink" supplement with 4 oz of water and feed this to your dog; the animal will quickly lick the bowl clean, enjoying the alkalinizing food.

Want proof that our modern-day diet is composed of too many acidifying foods? Just walk around any large supermarket and you will notice that the fresh fruit and vegetable section is, at maximum, 5–10 percent of the total area of the store. Color-coded fruit and vegetables are your primary alkalinizing foods.

Warning: When you shop, stay on the perimeter of a supermarket where fruit, vegetables, sprouts, herbs, flowers, fat-free plain yogurt, fat-free cottage cheese, free-range eggs, lean meats or fish, whole grains, and bins of legumes, seeds, and unsalted nuts can be found. Once you enter the aisles, you encounter an expensive array of modified, processed, highly packaged, acidifying foods that dissolve your teeth, nails, and bones—and harden your artery walls, heart tissues, and brain neurons. These foods look good, smell good, and taste good, but they carry a hefty hidden price tag. I call these foods the "foods of modern commerce."

Today a supermarket may contain 50,000 items, much of it processed foods made from acidifying refined grains, sugars, sweeteners, and cheap fats with annual North American sales of about $290 billion U.S.

IS DIETARY PROTEIN BENEFICIAL OR DETRIMENTAL TO BONE-BUILDING?

Protein is essential for the intestinal absorption of calcium, and protein is a major building block for new bone construction. Neither vitamin D3 nor K2 nor calcium can produce healthy bone mineralization without adequate supplies of lean protein.

Bone is a complex living structure comprised of cells, mineral crystals, and thick matrix proteins that, like glue, hold the entire bone together. In epidemiological studies, a lower intake of protein is associated with an increased risk of osteoporosis, according to the journal *Bone*. By weight, roughly one-third of our bone is a living, organic protein mix.

While adequate protein is essential to healthy bone-building, Harvard University's Mark Hegsted, Ph.D., writing in the *American Journal of Clinical Nutrition*, in 2001, reported that excessive protein from meat and grains greatly increased the net acidic load in the body by 50 percent, causing accelerated bone-breakdown. The researchers said, "Higher-protein diets increase circulating concentrations of anabolic (favorable) insulin-like growth hormone 1 (IGF-1), a recognized bone growth-promoting factor, if the protein's net acid load can be offset by eating more alkalinizing fruit and vegetables. Such diets would resemble that of our hunter-gatherer ancestors." The *American Journal of Clinical Nutrition*, in November 2005, reported that, "Higher supplemental calcium intake results in more absorbed calcium, which may help offset the urine losses induced by increased dietary animal protein."

In conclusion, the anabolic (favorable) impact of dietary protein on the skeleton is favorable if you are meeting your daily calcium requirements. Furthermore, if you consume a wide variety of colorful fruits and vegetables daily, the catabolic (unfavorable) acids produced from the protein will be properly buffered and you enhance bone-building. The researchers concluded that, "The balance between the amount of protein in the diet (anabolic effect) and the net acid load of the diet (catabolic effect) determines whether the diet supports bone-building or bone-breakdown." Protein is necessary. Simply neutralize its acidic effect by eating colorful produce and daily using a broad-spectrum, comprehensive bone-building supplement.

Whey isolate protein powder has an alkalinizing effect on the body and is a superior protein source to boost metabolic bone-building functions. Every morning, jumpstart your day with the one-minute power protein shake I describe in Chapter 10, as Bone-Building Tip 1.

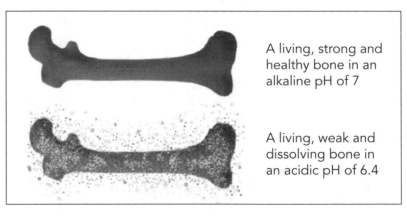

A living, strong and healthy bone in an alkaline pH of 7

A living, weak and dissolving bone in an acidic pH of 6.4

Figure 7.6: Bone Analysis

The Effects of Food on the Super-Critical Acid/Alkaline Biochemical Balance

Most Alkaline	Medium Alkaline	Low Alkaline	Foods	Low Acid	Medium Acid	Most Acid
broccoli cucumber cilantro oriental greens garlic onions kale spinach parsley sea vegetables greens+ "green drink"	bell pepper cauliflower parsnip endive ginger root sweet potato cabbage celery carrots asparagus	brussels sprouts beets, tops & roots tomatoes & tomato juice fresh peas dark lettuce all mushrooms fresh potato w/skin pumpkin squash tempeh	**Vegetables** **Beans** **Legumes** only use non-GMO foods	corn lentils peanuts w/skin organic peanut butter soy protein powder beans: kidney, lima, navy, pinto, white, black, soy peas: green, split & chick tofu (extra firm) edamame	salted peanut butter	processed soybeans salted & sweetened peanut butter

75% ← daily food choices, by volume, should ideally be → 25%

(Continue on page 194)

(Continued from page 193)

Most Alkaline	Medium Alkaline	Low Alkaline	Foods	Low Acid	Medium Acid	Most Acid
cantaloupe honeydew raisins nectarine raspberry watermelon fresh black cherries black olives in oil	apple avocado pink grapefruit lemons limes mangoes pear peach	pineapple apricot grapes blueberry strawberry blackberry papaya	**Fruits**	dry fruits natural figs dates prunes banana unsweetened canned fruit natural fruit juice unsweetened jams unsweetened preserves	olives, pickled sweetened fruit juice sweetened canned fruit sweetened jams sweetened preserves	cranberries sulfured dried fruit

	← 75%			Seasonings / Herbs / Spices · Beverages			25% →
Seasonings Herbs Spices	Celtic sea salt Antarctic sea salt miso & natto cayenne ashwagandha gotu kola ginkgo biloba baking soda (sodium bicarbonate)	cinnamon ginger dill, mint, peppermint turmeric rhodiola basil oregano licorice root Siberian ginseng	most herbs curry, mustard powder kola nut tamari milk thistle maca astragalus suma echinacea	tahini carob cocoa regular table salt	vanilla nutmeg mayonnaise ketchup		black pepper MSG soya sauce brewer's & nutritional yeast
Beverages	electron-rich alkaline water plasma activated water (PAW)	Teas: green, matcha green, ginger, rooibos, chamomile water ozonated water ionized water	dry red wine unsweetened almond milk distilled water beer (draft) or dark stout black coffee (organic)	unsweetened soy milk unsweetened rice milk black tea black coffee decaf coffee	coffee (milk & sugar)		alcoholic drinks soft drinks

75% ← daily food choices, by volume, should ideally be → 25%

(Continue on page 196)

(Continued from page 195)

Most Alkaline	Medium Alkaline	Low Alkaline	Foods	Low Acid	Medium Acid	Most Acid
bee pollen soy lecithin granules dairy-free probiotic cultures	aloe vera juice	whole oats quinoa wild rice millet & spelt plain hemp-protein powder	**Grains Cereals Other**	brown & basmati rice wheat & buckwheat kasha amaranth whole wheat & corn pasta whole grain bread	plain rice-protein powder rolled oats & oat bran rye white bread white pasta white rice	barley pastries cakes tarts cookies
pumpkin seeds almonds w/skin plain almond butter w/skin all sprouts wheat grass alfalfa grass barley grass	extra virgin olive oil borage oil & primrose oil chestnuts Brazil nuts light & dark flaxseeds macadamia nuts black currant oil	hazelnuts flaxseed & sea buckthorn oils hemp seeds & oil sesame seeds & oil sunflower seeds & oil fresh coconut & oil	**Nuts & Seeds Grasses and Sprouts Oils** only use cold-pressed oils	popcorn canola oil grape seed oil pine nuts safflower oil	cashews pecans walnuts	pistachios trans fatty acids acrylamides

75% (most ideal)						25% (least ideal)
human breast milk	wild, ultra-pure omega3 fish oil / CLA (conjugated linoleic acid)	cod liver oil	**Meats Fish & Fowl**	fish, turkey, venison, wild duck, seafood	chicken, lamb, pork, veal	beef, lobster
human breast milk	dairy probiotic cultures, whey protein isolate powder	soft goat cheese, fresh goat milk	**Dairy Eggs**	cow's milk, cream, yogurt, butter, buttermilk, white of chicken eggs	soy cheese & soft cheese, ice cream, whole chicken eggs	processed cheese, hard cheese, yolk of chicken eggs
	blackstrap molasses (unsulfured)	stevia, brown rice syrup, pure maple syrup, unpasteurized honey	**Sweeteners**	commercial honey	corn syrup & fructose, high-fructose corn syrup, sugar	artificial sweeteners
		apple cider vinegar	**Vinegar**	rice vinegar	balsamic vinegar	white vinegar

daily food choices, by volume, should ideally be 75% ↔ 25%

BREAKTHROUGH LIFESAVING
MEDICINE BASED ON pH

Dr. Stephen Russell, a cancer specialist at the Mayo Clinic, knows how to use pH in a novel approach to seek, find, and destroy cancer cells. The one characteristic of a malignant tumor is that it continues to divide extremely well with little or no oxygen in an acidic, anaerobic environment—the same acidic environment that bacteria and viruses need to replicate.

Using this knowledge, Dr. Russell and another cancer researcher, Dr. Kenneth Kinzler of Johns Hopkins Hospital's Kimmel Cancer Center, are rehabilitating bad bugs such as viruses and bacteria (which operate well in an acidic, anaerobic environment) into therapeutic, lifesaving good bugs! Using the basic tools of molecular biology, Dr. Russell and Dr. Kinzler are reprogramming and transforming common microbes like the clostridium, salmonella, and C. botulinum bacteria or the Epstein-Barr virus (EBV) to attack a cancer cell, divide furiously, penetrate the malignant cell, continue to replicate, then produce deadly natural toxins and destroy the cell from within. They have learned to attach molecular tracking proteins to the microbe to make sure that once it is set free, it does not deviate from its therapeutic mission of targeting cancer cells.

These are good microbes to use because even if the microbe did go awry, the infection could be easily controlled with antibiotics or antiviral medications. Other microbiologists are modifying strains of viruses and bacteria to become ideal vehicles for delivering potent cancer drugs. Dr. Russell and Dr. Eva Galanis constructed a measles virus that recognizes and targets a mutation often found in brain tumor cells but never in normal cells.

More than 95 percent of the population is infected with EBV. Dr. Cliona Rooney, an immunovirologist at the Texas Medical Center, has retrained EBV to recognize, target, and form identical protein bonds with three different types of cancer—throat cancer, Hodgkin's disease, and non-Hodgkin's lymphoma. This cutting-edge idea is to have a therapeutically modified bacteria or virus exploit something unique to the cancer cell. The easiest method is to use rehabilitated, altered microbes like clostridium to replicate only in the oxygen-starved, acidic, anaerobic depths of a tumor. Once inside the cancer cell, the bacterium releases its toxins, which quickly eat through the malignant growth to the acidic interior of a cancer cell. This therapy has been tested only in mice, but with impressive results.

The bacterium salmonella and the measles virus also have the ability to quickly zero in on tumor cells. In a small pilot study conducted at the Mary Crowley Medical Research Center in Dallas, two of three patients given the altered, rehabilitated salmonella had impressive results. These studies point to something more exciting.

Rehabilitating, retraining and re-outfitting bad bugs to be therapeutic, natural chemotherapy "good guys" attacking a malignant tumor at its acidic, anaerobic core is good mind-body medicine. The technology exists to make it an achievable goal.
—Jesse Lynn Hanley, M.D., author of *Tired of Being Tired*

Cellular biologists are learning to cover the microbes with a protein coating that cloaks them like a stealth bomber and renders them invisible to immune cell radar long enough so that they can deliver a lethal, natural "toxic drop" on a cancer cell's periphery, then eat into the acidic core of the cancer cell and destroy it. One thing is certain: Medical research will undergo greater, more captivating changes during the next decade than in the last 500 years; we are going to vastly expand both our mental and physical horizons. In the meantime, most researchers are keeping their pH slightly alkaline—and so should you.

> Fifteen minutes before breakfast use a food-based "green drink" bone-building supplement because you need an alkalinizing power shift to imitate your ancestor's nutrient-rich diet.

The main message is to keep your body slightly alkaline by eating lots of colorful vegetables, salads, herbs, spices, "green drinks," and fresh fruit, which allows enzymes, peptide chaperones, hormones, neurotransmitters, and neuropeptides to operate efficiently.

You can incorporate dietary and lifestyle choices that boost and balance your alkalinity, good mood, vibrant energy, immune system, bone mineral density (BMD), and strength to experience your fulfilled and dynamic best self all life long.

This is the kind of high-impact change we can all benefit from.

Chapter 8

Smart Bone-Building Food Choices

Your diet has a significant effect on the health of your 206 bones and 143 joints. This makes sense, since the biological processes by which the micro-architecture of bone is constantly being dissolved and rebuilt involves nutrients, vitamins, and minerals extracted from the bloodstream. Surprisingly, achieving the optimum dietary intake of essential bone-building nutrients may not be as easy as simply eating a well-balanced diet.

Hippocrates, the father of modern medicine, in 500 BC, said, "Let food be your medicine, and let medicine be your food." While our daily intake of some nutrients like calcium and magnesium is woefully low, others, such as phosphorus, are in excess. Both dietary deficiencies and excesses present significant problems for healthy bone maintenance.

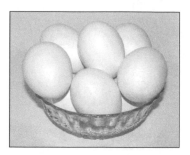

Figure 8.1: Nature Needs Calcium for Structure

IS YOUR BONE BANK ACCOUNT RUNNING LOW?

There is a real problem with the average person not getting enough daily nutrients. Your body is always monitoring your bloodstream to keep all nutrients, like calcium, at just the right levels so it is available equally to all cells. Your bones are a "bone bank account" that can store extra calcium reserves. When the calcium in your bloodstream dips even a little bit, your body withdraws calcium from the "bone bank account."

> Thirty-one million people today suffer from low bone mass in North America, and by the year 2020, that number is expected to rise to 62 million.

Obviously, if this continues you end up with low bone mineral density and weak bones until you start to take in more calcium than you are losing, and invest more calcium back into your "bone bank account." But as we know, calcium cannot do its critical work alone. In order to do its job effectively, it needs the entire bone-building team of vitamin B6, vitamin B9, vitamin B12, "friendly" probiotic cultures, vitamin D3, non-acidic vitamin C, vitamin K2, and the trace minerals boron, magnesium, calcium, silicon, copper, and zinc. It is normal to lose some calcium daily in our excretions (both urine and stool) as well as our sweat and through our lungs when we breathe. Therefore, we need to consume enough of these essential nutrients daily through supplements and through natural food sources to make up for these losses. The foods you eat today and the supplements you use daily determine your future bone quantity, quality, and strength.

CALCIUM

People often find it difficult to consume their daily requirement of calcium in the form of food. Some have trouble digesting lactose (lactose maldigestion or lactose intolerance), the sugar in milk, and find that dairy-based foods upset their stomach. Others find it difficult to eat enough calcium-rich foods. For those with lactose maldigestion or lactose intolerance, some dairy-based foods such as yogurt cause less discomfort. Lactose pills taken before consumption of dairy-based foods can curtail gastrointestinal symptoms. If you have lactose intolerance or do not otherwise consume enough dairy products, bone-building supplements containing calcium will help you achieve your daily requirement.

Calcium is needed for:

- strong bones, healthy teeth, and clear nails
- reducing the risk of colon cancer
- enhancing learning and reducing ADD and ADHD
- achieving deep, sound restorative sleep
- proper weight management

A Note on Soft Drinks and Calcium

Soft drinks are high in phosphoric acid and sugar, making them very acidifying. Phosphoric acid requires calcium and potassium to neutralize or buffer its corrosive acids, and pulls calcium out of the bones to accomplish this buffering action. The result is that calcium is excreted with the phosphoric acid. To remedy this, the parathyroid gland restores calcium balance in the blood by pulling calcium from bone. Consequently, anything highly acidic like soft drinks can directly lead to osteoporosis and raises the risk for fracture.

The average North American drinks 56 gallons of soda a year, which is equivalent to 600, 12 oz cans. Each sugar-sweetened soda containing 10 tsps of acidifying sugar and each diet soda containing acidifying non-calorie sugar substitutes are providing only empty calories while replacing more nutritious drinks.

Part of the problem is that many adolescents and adults who drink lots of sodas and colas also drink very little milk and eat very few dairy products like fat-free organic, plain yogurt, and other calcium-dense foods. A cola has a pH of 2.5 and is so acidic it could kill you if your body does not have enough alkaline buffering minerals like calcium, magnesium, or potassium, which form into bicarbonates in your bloodstream, acting like "acid sponges."

Other Nutrients Influence the Calcium Balance

The calcium contained in food we eat is digested in the stomach, then moved into the small intestine where it is absorbed into the blood for use by the body. Certain foods can decrease the absorption of calcium. These include *caffeine, wheat fiber, phytates, oxalates,* and *supplemental iron.* Excessive caffeine should be avoided for many reasons, though moderate caffeine consumption is not detrimental to health.

Iron pills or vitamins containing iron should not be taken with calcium since calcium and iron interfere with each other's absorption.

In contrast, wheat fiber is an important part of the diet as it might help maintain lower cholesterol levels and aid colon health maintenance. If you add supplemental fiber, try to get your calcium-dense foods at a different time. Foods containing phytates include beans, peas, seeds, nuts, and cereal grains.

Oxalates are found in spinach, sweet potato, rhubarb, Swiss chard, and beans. There is no reason from the perspective of the skeleton to avoid consumption of these products, however, since they have important nutrient value and an otherwise adequate calcium intake will be able to overcome any small influence of these nutrients on calcium absorption. For example, the calcium from spinach is not well absorbed; however, any other calcium eaten with the spinach will be well absorbed.

Tip: Squeeze fresh lemon juice on any foods containing oxalates to break down the oxalic acid.

Other foods that influence calcium balance in the body include salt and protein. Excessive consumption of these products might increase the amount of calcium excreted in the urine.

How to Read Labels for Calcium Content

The calcium content of foods varies widely upon grow-ing conditions and the amount of calcium added to fortified foods. Reading the food label is an easy way to find out how much calcium is in one serving of a food. Food labels may list calcium in milligrams or as a percentage of Daily Value. To find the calcium content (mg per serving), do the following calculation:

If the calcium per serving on the label says 20% calcium, simply drop the % and add a "0." For ex-ample, 20% calcium equals 200 mg of calcium.

In general, many North Americans are eating too much table salt and meat protein, so reducing intake is likely warranted for purposes completely separate from bone health, such as heart and blood vessel health.

In the rural regions of China, osteoporosis is rare despite half the calcium intake of North Americans. What is the key to understanding this paradox? It all gets back to alkalinity.

Our bodies place maintenance of bloodstream cal-cium well above the maintenance of bone strength. The body is preprogrammed to sacrifice its skeleton to maintain blood calcium. Protein is made of amino acids and phosphorus, which create an acidic environment in the bloodstream. If we have enough calcium, mag-nesium, potassium, and sodium in our systems from eating plenty of fresh fruits, salads, and vegetables, our bodies make alkalizing salts like potassium bicar-bonate. If we do not have enough of these minerals, the body dissolves calcium from our bones, leading to urinary calcium loss. For example, eating double your necessary daily protein from animal sources increases urinary calcium by 50 percent.

Calcium and Magnesium for a Good Night's Sleep

A lack of calcium and magnesium can cause you to wake up after a few hours and not be able to return to sleep. Calcium is needed to help promote sleep by calming the nervous system. Insufficient amounts of calcium and magnesium can cause nervous tension, fatigue, and muscle cramping, which can interfere with your sleep. Low levels of calcium and magnesium in the diet may be a contributing factor to restless leg syndrome. Calcium, combined with magnesium, relaxes muscles and improves deep sleep patterns.

Getting Calcium from Food

It is often possible, if wise food choices are made, to obtain the optimal calcium intake from food. These include milk, yogurt, and cheese as well as cheese-containing mixed dishes. The soy-based and rice-based milks, yogurts, tofu, and cheeses are available fortified to contain amounts of calcium similar to those of cow's milk-based dairy products. Surprisingly so, sea vegetables are the richest source of calcium.

Canned fish products with bones (salmon, sardines) also contain a generous amount of calcium; fresh fish fillets without bones, however, are not a significant source. Some vegetables contain significant amounts of calcium, particularly bok choy, dandelion, turnip and mustard greens, kale, artichokes, and broccoli. Many other foods contain small amounts of calcium, including baked beans, oranges, almonds, and hummus. Remarkably, four dried figs contain 112 mg of bioavailable calcium.

A list of the calcium content of certain foods is provided.

Food Sources of Calcium Serving Size Calcium in mg		
SEAFOOD	Serving Size	mg
Mackerel (canned, with bones)	3 oz	260
Oysters	3 oz	80
Perch	3 oz	115
Salmon (canned, with bones)	3 oz	200
Sardines (canned, with bones)	3 oz	340
Shrimp (canned)	3 oz	95
VEGETABLES and FRUIT	Serving Size	mg
Acorn squash	1 cup	90
Bok choy (cooked)	1 cup	230
Broccoli (cooked)	1 cup	160
Brussels sprouts	1 cup	55
Collard greens	1 cup	350
Dried figs	4 figs	112
Kale (cooked)	1 cup	180
Mustard greens	1 cup	160
Okra (cooked)	1 cup	220
Orange	1	55
Rutabaga (cooked)	1 cup	100
Turnip greens	1 cup	230

NUTS	Serving Size	mg
Almonds	3.5 oz	266
Brazil nuts	3.5 oz	176
Hazelnuts	3.5 oz	188
Peanuts	3.5 oz	58
Sesame and flaxseeds	1 tbsp	90
Walnuts	3.5 oz	94
CALCIUM-FORTIFIED BEVERAGES	Serving Size	mg
Grapefruit juice, fortified	8 oz	400
Mineral water	4 cups	200
Orange juice, fortified	8 oz	350
Rice milk, fortified	1 cup	240
Soy milk, fortified	1 cup	160
YOGURT	Serving Size	mg
Frozen, low-fat or non-fat	1 cup	300
Fruit, low-fat	1 cup	314
Plain, fat-free	1 cup	452
Plain, low-fat	1 cup	415
MILK	Serving Size	mg
Buttermilk	1 cup	285
Chocolate	1 cup	280
Condensed, sweetened	1 cup	837
Evaporated	1 cup	329
Evaporated, non-fat	1 cup	329
Half and half	1 cup	254
Non-fat, dry	1 cup	1,508
Non-fat, skim	1 cup	300
Sour cream	1 cup	268
Whipping cream, light	1 cup	166
Whipping cream, heavy	1 cup	154
Whole	1 cup	291
Whole, dry	1 cup	1,168

(Continue on page 210)

(Continued from page 209)

Food Sources of Calcium *Serving Size Calcium in mg*		
CHEESE	Serving Size	mg
American	1 oz	195
Blue cheese	1 oz	150
Brie	1 oz	52
Camembert	1 oz	110
Cheddar	1 oz	204
Cottage, low-fat, 1%	1 oz	137
Edam	1 oz	207
Feta	1 oz	140
Fontina	1 oz	156
Goat cheese	1 oz	85
Gouda	1 oz	198
Gruyère	1 oz	287
Monterey Jack	1 oz	212
Mozzarella	1 oz	183
Muenster	1 oz	203
Parmesan, fresh	1 oz	336
Parmesan, grated	1 oz	168
Ricotta, part skim	1 cup	669
Romano	1 oz	302
Soft cheese	1 oz	130
Swiss	1 oz	250

VITAL VITAMIN D3

Vitamin D3 not only helps with calcium absorption, it also aids in the biochemical process by which calcium turns into bone. In fact, when you read the fine print in scientific studies of fractures and calcium supplements, the only research showing reductions in fractures are studies where calcium was combined with vitamin D3!

We get vitamin D3 from two sources: diet (including supplements) and sun exposure.

Vitamin D3 is needed for:

- proper calcium absorption in the intestine
- superior development of the micro-architecture of bone
- prevention against prostate and breast cancers
- support of the parathyroid gland, responsible for monitoring bone development
- improving treatment outcomes in people already diagnosed with cancer

Vitamin D3 and the Sun: A Deeper Look

Special cells in our skin produce vitamin D3 when they're activated by ultraviolet light. A young person who spends part of the day outdoors in the summer can get all the vitamin D3 they need from the sun. But this is much more difficult for older people. If a 65-year-old mother and her 35-year old daughter take a 10-minute walk on a sunny day, the mother's skin will manufacture only a third of the amount of vitamin D3 that her daughter's does. To make matters worse, the angle of the sun's rays changes in the winter, and in many parts of the country even a sunny day doesn't provide the necessary stimulation for our skin cells. If you live in an area that's far enough north for snow, you probably don't get enough vitamin D3 during the winter. Several studies have shown that bone density drops slowly through the winter, reaching a low point in late spring. The loss can amount to 3 or 4 percent. My advice is to supplement daily with vitamin D3. Sunlight is too weak in all of Canada and the northern U.S. for vitamin D3 synthesis from October to March.

Vitamin D3 and Food

The need for vitamin D3 increases as we get older. Most adults get 100–200 IU per day in their diet. That's enough for young people (who also get vitamin D3 from sun exposure), but it's well under the higher needs for those over 30.

Vitamin D3 Requirements for Men and Women	
Age	Daily Recommended Intake in international units and micrograms (mcg) equivalent 40 IU = 1 mcg
Birth to age 50	1,000 IU or 25 mcg
51–70	1,000 IU or 25 mcg
71 and older	2,000 IU or 50 mcg

The problem is that few foods naturally contain significant amounts of vitamin D3. The best sources are cold saltwater fish and other seafood, like salmon, halibut, herring, tuna, Atlantic mackerel, oysters, and shrimp. The liver and oil from these fish are extremely high in vitamin D3. Some mushrooms are also good sources, including shiitakes and morels.

Because this vitamin is so important, a committee of the American Medical Association recommended in 1957 that milk be fortified with 400 IU of vitamin D3 per quart. This requirement has been mandated by the federal government ever since. Vitamin D3 is also added to some fortified cereals and to many calcium supplements.

The year 2005 produced stunning research findings suggesting that vitamin D3 has applications in promoting bone strength. Moreover, scientists are examining the role of vitamin D3 to reduce the risk of no fewer than 17 different types of cancer, ranging from colon, breast, and prostate cancers to ovarian, renal, and bladder cancer. Furthermore, researchers believe vitamin D3 may even improve treatment outcomes in people already diagnosed with cancer according to the *Journal of Nutrition*, February 2005; the *Cancer Journal*, September 2005; and *Endocrinology*, April 2005.

> **Tip:** Use a high-quality bone-builder supplement daily that contains 800 IU of natural vitamin D3.

VITAMIN K

Vitamin K1, or phylloquinone, is found in any green vegetable containing the green pigment chlorophyll and its water-soluble derivative, chlorophyllin. Vitamin K1, in the presence of "friendly" probiotic bacteria in the intestines, is converted into the more biologically active form called K2, or menaquinones. K2 is found in egg yolks, butter, and fermented soy foods. K2 helps the body make and activate two critical proteins, osteocalcin and matrix G1a, in a biochemical process called gamma-carboxylation. Osteocalcin and matrix G1a are calcium-binding proteins, absolutely essential to guide calcium into the osteoblast cells of bones, make strong bone tissues, and prevent osteoporosis.

Vitamin K2 (like vitamin D) is produced in the body by certain healthy intestinal bacteria.

Vitamin K is needed for:

- activating two critical proteins responsible for delivering calcium into the bone
- actively keeping calcium from calcifying in soft tissues like the heart and arteries
- the formation of two bone-building proteins, osteocalcin and matrix G1a

Food Sources of Vitamin K	
Asparagus	Green peas
Bok choy	Green tea
Cereals	Liver
Eggs	Meat
Green beans	Milk
"Green drinks"	Oats
Green, leafy vegetables	Whole wheat

MAGNESIUM

Magnesium is a bone-builder. It is critical for:

- helping transport calcium in and out of bone
- increasing the activity of vitamin D3, which enhances calcium absorption
- regulating the parathyroid gland
- activating bone-building osteoblasts

There is strong evidence that magnesium depletion contributes to osteoporosis. In fact, in some cases magnesium may be even more important than calcium. The appropriate calcium to magnesium ratio is 1.5 to 1. This means that if you are getting 500 mg of calcium at each meal from a bone-building food source, you should also be getting 300 mg of magnesium from your diet, and this is especially true if you already have osteoporosis. If you have a heart condition or arthritis, you may need even more magnesium, so be sure to ask your health care provider what the appropriate calcium/magnesium ratio is for you.

As with all mineral supplements, I believe that aspartate forms of magnesium are the best. A chelated mineral is one that has undergone a procedure that involves binding it to an amino acid or carbohydrate so that it becomes easier to absorb. The evidence shows that magnesium asparate is better absorbed and used by the body than inorganic magnesium oxide. Magnesium aspartate also helps prevent calcium-stone formation in the kidneys. High single doses of magnesium more than 350 mg may cause diarrhea, so it is better to take several smaller doses with food throughout the day if you specifically need more magnesium.

Food Sources of Magnesium	
Blackstrap molasses	Legumes: soybeans, dried beans, peas, edamame
Brown rice	Nuts: almonds, Brazil, cashew
Buckwheat	Seeds: pumpkin, sesame, sunflower, flax, hemp
Corn and rye	
Dandelion greens	Wheat germ and amaranth
Dark-green vegetables: spinach, lettuce	Whole-grain cereals
Figs	

Magnesium is one of the minerals that make up bone, and it's also important for many chemical reactions, including conduction of nerve impulses to the heart and other parts of the body.

Research indicates that people whose diets are rich in magnesium have denser bones. Magnesium is as important as calcium in the prevention and treatment of osteoporosis. Not only does magnesium contribute to bone mineral mass, but it is critical for the proper function of vitamin D3. Magnesium has been clearly established to protect against cardiovascular disease.

Some calcium supplements contain magnesium as well as vitamin D3. I urge you to think of magnesium as yet another important benefit of a diet that includes plenty of fruits and vegetables and whole grains. Most people don't get nearly as much magnesium as they should. The daily recommended intake for magnesium is 320 mg per day for women and 429 mg for men, but the average actual intake is only around 250 mg per day. Though this seems like a small deficit, it contributes to osteoporosis. I recommend 750 mg per day.

Magnesium is an important team player, with a role in regulating active calcium transport. A two-year study of postmenopausal women supplemented with magnesium showed significant protection from osteoporosis and greater bone mineral density.

You can easily increase your consumption of magnesium because it's contained in so many healthy foods. Among the best sources are potatoes, seeds, nuts, legumes, and whole grains (most of the magnesium is in the husk and germ). Magnesium is also found in chlorophyll, so any dark-green vegetable—romaine lettuce, spinach, kale—contains a good supply. The darker the color, the better. Other good sources are bananas, oranges, and tomatoes.

Magnesium has a role in the production of a bone hormone called parathyroid hormone (PTH). When magnesium is low, less PTH is released. Normal levels of PTH cause bone to be produced, but high levels of PTH cause calcium to be leached from bone. Scientists agree that more research is necessary to pin down the exact role of magnesium when it comes to bone health.

POTASSIUM

Potassium is the latest nutrient with research-proven benefits for bone. Katherine Tucker's nutritional research on Farmingham Heart study participants found that men and women whose diet is high in potassium have denser bones in their spines and hips; one other study has documented the same effect. The likely reason: Potassium contributes to the proper acid balance in the blood, so the body doesn't need to draw calcium from the skeleton for this purpose. Potassium serves us in other ways: It's needed for proper fluid balance in our bodies, for conduction of nerve impulses, and for muscle contractions.

Potassium is needed for:

- maintaining an alkaline pH
- regulating blood pressure
- optimizing efficient bone-repair
- normalizing heart rhythms
- regulating the body's water balance

The current guidelines call for 4,700 mg a day. In Dr. Tucker's study, a woman's diet was considered high in potassium if she consumed 3,500–6,000 mg per day. That's not difficult to do if you eat plenty of fruits—especially oranges and cantaloupe—and vegetables.

Dairy products contain moderate amounts of potassium. So far there's no research supporting the need to supplement potassium for bone-building. This is likely because a single cup of sweet potato has 950 mg, four figs boast 540 mg, a cup of cantaloupe 1,500 mg, and a glass of OJ 450 mg!

Potassium is remarkably effective at lowering blood pressure—and even a 1–2 percent reduction translates into a reduced risk of strokes. University of Mississippi physiologist Dr. David B. Young says, "Unless you have kidney disease, potassium is one of those things, like love and money, that you just can't get too much of."

Food Sources of Potassium	
All seeds and nuts	Milk
All soy	Orange juice
Apples	Poultry
Bananas	Prunes
Cantaloupe	Sweet potato
Cheese	Yogurt
Fish	

VITAMIN C

We all know how important vitamin C is. Whole books have been written about the almost magical qualities of this water-soluble vitamin, which is able to boost the immune system, help heal wounds, and provide antioxidant properties that prevent cell damage by neutralizing free radicals. Some studies even suggest that people who eat a lot of foods high in vitamin C lower their risk of cancer, heart disease, and age-related macular degeneration (AMD).

Vitamin C:

- is an antioxidant
- combats the process of oxidation, which is a major factor in the aging of our bodies
- keeps our skin, eyes, and gums healthy
- helps ward off infection
- appears to play an important role in collagen production, the first step in bone formation

Most people get around 70 mg per day, slightly above the current recommendation of 60 mg per day. However, there's evidence that people whose diet contains more vitamin C have better bones. The best source is citrus fruit. But other fruits (especially bananas, cantaloupe, and strawberries) and some vegetables (including peppers, broccoli, asparagus, cauliflower, tomatoes, and sweet potatoes) also contain significant amounts. With all those outrageously deliciously options, it's easy to get plenty of vitamin C from food.

When it comes to bone health, vitamin C is essential for the formation of the cement-like substance that forms the internal supporting structure of the bone. The recommended dietary allowance is 125 mg a day for adult men and 90 mg a day for adult women, but I find this recommendation low; I personally use 1,200 mg a day.

Food Sources of Vitamin C	
All sprouts	Citrus fruits: oranges, grapefruit, lemons, limes
Broccoli	
Cabbage	Red peppers
Cantaloupe	Tomatoes

MANGANESE

Manganese is another trace element that we need in very small amounts for proper nutrition. No official daily allowance has been established, but 2–5 mg is the National Research Council's recommended average adult requirement. The best natural sources are whole-grain cereals, nuts, green leafy vegetables, peas, and beans.

Manganese:

- is needed for normal bone structure
- helps to eliminate fatigue
- aids in muscle reflexes
- reduces nervous irritability

It appears that manganese is critical to the development of cartilage and bone. New research has shown that manganese deficiency seems to increase bone breakdown, while at the same time it decreases new bone mineralization. The opposite has also been shown to be true: bone-breakdown decreases with higher blood serum levels of manganese. One study in particular showed that women with osteoporosis had only one quarter of the manganese levels of women who did not have osteoporosis.

Food Sources of Manganese	
All nuts and seeds	Red Meats
Fish	Spinach
Legumes: dried beans, peas	Whole grains

You may find this interesting. Manganese has replaced lead in gasoline. This means that there is more manganese in the air as a kind of pollutant. There should, as a result of this, be more manganese in foods, so that a deficiency is less likely now than ever.

ZINC

Researchers consider zinc loss a marker for osteoporosis because studies show that postmenopausal women often have a significant increase in the loss of zinc, and these are the women most susceptible to developing osteoporosis.

Zinc is responsible for:

- producing both osteoblasts and osteoclasts
- encouraging bone to heal
- boosting vitamin D function
- stimulating the release of hormones
- metabolizing protein

We have about 2 gm of zinc in our body, most of which is found in our bone tissue, eyes, liver, and, in males, prostate. Zinc is important because it plays an essential role in DNA and protein synthesis, and it is necessary for the formation of osteoblasts and osteoclasts, meaning it influences the turnover of bone.

There are some foods that inhibit the absorption of zinc. They are brown rice, whole-grain cereals and breads, wheat bran, and legumes (soy beans, dried beans, and peas). Try to take your zinc at meals when you are not eating these foods.

Food Sources of Zinc	
Beef	Oysters
Cheese	Pork
Chicken	Seeds: pumpkin, sesame, flax, and sunflower
Eggs	
Lamb	Whole grains, bran, wheat, wheat germ
Legumes: dried beans, peas	Zinc-fortified cereals: bran flakes, oatmeal,raisin bran and rye
Lobster	
Milk	
Nuts: cashews, peanuts, pecans	

BORON

Boron may mimic the action of estrogen and testoster-one, hormones that protect bone health. In one report, men and women lost calcium and magnesium from their bodies when they were made boron deficient, and retained those minerals on a boron-supplemented diet; they also manufactured more estrogen and testosterone when on boron supplementation, which is extremely beneficial, especially after the age of 34 when natural estrogen and testosterone levels begin to decline. Estrogen in women and testosterone in men are hormones directly related to maximum bone-building. In another study, vitamin D3 status improved in boron-deficient men and women after they received boron.

Boron is needed for:

- strong, efficient bone-building
- assisting calcium and vitamin D3 to function at optimum
- the relief of osteoarthritis

- proper parathyroid gland metabolism
- raising low levels of estrogen in women and testosterone in men

In 2003 and 2004, the journals *Prostate* and *Oncology* published studies by Dr. Gallardo-Williams and Dr. Y. Cui and colleagues at UCLA revealing that men with the highest boron intake reduced "Their prostate cancer risk by 54 percent compared to those with the lowest boron intake—prostate-specific androgen levels plummeted by an average of 87 percent!" There is a patented natural complex of food-sourced boron that is more bioavailable than any other form of boron. The name of this boron is OsteoBoron. OsteoBoron has been the subject of clinical studies demonstrating its efficacy in the support of healthy bones and joints.

Food Sources of Boron	
Almond butter	Legumes (cooked): black-eyed peas, lima beans, kidney beans, pinto beans
Almonds	
Apples (red)	Oranges
Applesauce	Parsley
Avocado	Peaches
Broccoli	Peanut butter
Carrots	Peanuts
Celery	Pears
Cherries	Plums
Dry red wine	Prune Juice
Flaxseed	Prunes
Grape juice	Raisins
Grapes	Spinach
Hemp seed	Squash
	Strawberries

COPPER

Copper is an essential trace mineral that recently has been found to be important in maintaining bone health. This was discovered when professional basketball star Bill Walton kept breaking bones even though he was a young, healthy athlete. When doctors analyzed his diet, they found it lacked the trace minerals zinc, selenium, copper, and manganese. When he started taking supplements of these minerals, along with calcium, his condition was cured. Although we are not sure exactly how copper works in bone health, we do know that it is an aid in the formation of collagen for bone and connective tissue. Inadequate levels of copper, as well as manganese, have been associated with osteoporosis. The total amount in the adult body is 100–150 mg. Many essential enzyme systems are dependent on traces of copper.

> **Copper Deficiency:** The average diet contains only 50 percent of the necessary copper. One study found that all segments of the population have a copper deficiency ranging from 50–59 percent.

Copper is needed for:

- effective iron absorption
- converting the body's iron into hemoglobin
- assisting the amino acid tyrosine to support the thyroid gland
- superior bone strength and density
- efficient, daily bone repair

Food Sources of Copper		
All seeds	Lamb	Peanuts with skins
Brazil nuts	Legumes	Pork
Cereals	Liver	Seafood
Filberts	Oysters	Walnuts

SILICA OR SILICON

Herbalists have long used a silicon-rich plant called horsetail (*Equisetum arvense*) to heal bones. In animals, silicon deficiency causes bone defects. Dietary silicon is absorbed as orthosilicic acid, which has recently been shown to stimulate the synthesis of collagen type 1 (the kind found in bone matrix) and to induce characteristic osteoblast enzymes in osteoblast-like cells. In a recent small retrospective study, men and women who received silicon had significantly increased bone mineral density in the femur.

Silicon is the most abundant mineral on earth. We don't know much about how it actually works in the body, but we do know that it is abundant in our stronger tissues such as nails, hair, teeth, tendons, arteries, skin, connective tissue, and collagen. Bone collagen increases with silicon supplementation.

Silicon:

- strengthens our connective tissue matrix by cross-reinforcing our strands of protein collagen
- appears to increase bone mineralization when our calcium levels are low
- seems to initiate the calcification process in the bone, thereby keeping our bones strong and flexible

The human body contains approximately 7 gm of silicon, which is present in various tissues and body fluids.

Food Sources of Silicon	
Barley	Leeks
Beans, peas, legumes	Mother's milk
Bell peppers	Nuts and seeds
Brown rice	Oats
Cucumbers	Onions
Fruits (especially the skins)	Parsnips
Green leafy vegetables	Whole grains

VITAMIN B12 (COBALAMIN)

Vitamins play a different but equally essential role in healthy bone-building. There are necessary catalysts in various biochemical reactions involved in new bone formation. B12, another water-soluble vitamin, is on the list of essential nutrients for good bone health. Without adequate B12, our osteoblasts can't do their job. B12 is not found in plant foods, and sometimes vegetarians can develop a deficiency in this vitamin. It plays an essential role in red blood cell formation, cell metabolism, and nerve function. It is estimated that 10–30 percent of adults over 50 have a B12 deficiency because they can't absorb food-bound vitamin B12.

Large amounts of B12 are stored in the liver, so it can take years for a deficiency to show up. People who have pernicious anemia or who have had gastrointestinal surgery may require injections of B12 or sublingual methylcobalamin or hydroxycobalamin, the forms of B12 that I prefer.

B12 is needed for:

- breaking down homocysteine, lowering the risk of osteoporosis
- lowering the risk of heart disease
- abundant sustained energy
- a healthy nervous system
- improved concentration, memory, and balance

Food Sources of Vitamin B12	
Beans, peas, legumes	Nuts and seeds
Cheese	Organ meats
Dairy products	Poultry
Eggs	Shellfish
Fish	Some fortified cereals
Lentils	Tempeh and Miso
Meat	Turkey

VITAMIN B9 (FOLIC ACID/FOLATE)

Folic acid is the synthetic form of folate, a member of a vitamin B complex. Government agencies have been supportive that pregnant women or nursing mothers should receive 400 mcg of folic acid a day to protect babies at the time of conception and early pregnancy for neural-tube defects such as spina bifida. The best natural sources are egg and yolk, cantaloupe, apricot, pumpkins, avocadoes, beans, deep-green leafy vegetables, carrots, and liver. Folic acid is found in fortified cereals, fortified breads, and supplements. It is another water-soluble vitamin, and it is important in red blood cell formation, protein metabolism, growth, and cell division. It is also extremely important to the developing fetus in pregnant women and, surprisingly, to optimal bone-building.

Vitamin B9 is needed for:

- formation of red blood cells in the bone marrow
- efficient protein metabolism
- protecting against birth defects
- lifelong bone-repair and bone-building
- healthier looking skin

Food Sources of Vitamin B9	
Beans	Nuts
Eggs	Organ meats
Fish	Poultry
Lentils	Shellfish
Meat	Some fortified cereals
Miso	Tempeh, extra firm tofu

LYCOPENE

In September 2004, the medical journal *Urological Oncology* published a study of 20 men with prostate cancer in which each man received 10 mg of lycopene (from red tomatoes) for three months. No other treatment was given. Ten of the men reduced their prostate-specific androgen (PSA) by 50 percent and the study concluded, "Lycopene therapy appears to be effective and safe in the treatment of hormone-refractory prostate cancer."

Dr. V.A. Rao, Ph.D., Professor Emeritus, Department of Nutritional Sciences, University of Toronto, Faculty of Medicine, has studied the antioxidant capabilities of lycopene in detail, and he highly recommends 7 mg a day as a minimum for men and women as a preventative and for those living with chronic diseases. This recommendation can be extended in support of favorable osteoblast cell functioning and superior bone-building health based on the finding of Dr. Leticia Rao, Ph.D., Director of the Calcium Research Laboratory at St. Michael's Hospital.

Lycopene is needed for:

- an antioxidant in bone tissue, reducing inflammation
- an impressive antioxidant against harmful ultra-violet rays
- preventing macular degeneration
- preventing gum disease and the loss of teeth
- protecting against atherosclerosis

ISOFLAVONES

Recent research has demonstrated that isoflavones are found in legumes such as the soybean, but are actually most abundant in the Asian herb *kudzu*. Isoflavones have been noted to prevent hot flashes in women, lower total cholesterol levels, and provide protection against both heart disease and cancer. The latest research has shown that isoflavones support optimum bone-building efficiency by both lowering inflammation in the bone-building osteoblast cells and acting as natural antioxidants in those same cells. Isoflavones have also been used in the Orient for centuries to prevent hangovers and reduce the desire for alcohol! Research suggests that both men and women consume 90 mg of isoflavones daily to support optimum bone-building.

Isoflavones are needed for:

- optimum bone-building efficiency
- a potent antioxidant in bone-building cells
- reducing inflammation in bone-building cells
- protecting against both heart disease and cancer
- reducing the desire for alcohol

Isoflavones are naturally occurring in fermented soy products. Supermarkets and natural food stores carry an increasing variety of soy products. The five organic soy products rich in isoflavones that I highly recommend that you eat are:

1. soy milk, the unsweetened liquid from soybeans
2. extra-firm tofu, the soy equivalent of firm cottage cheese
3. unsalted roasted soy nuts, which can be eaten as a snack
4. tempeh, firmer than tofu with a delicious nutty flavor, is a fermented patty made from the soybean
5. edamame, my favorite product, are young, sweet, delicious Japanese soybeans that are steamed in their pods

IPRIFLAVONE

Ipriflavone is a synthetic derivative of isoflavones, available over the counter without a doctor's prescription. It is considered a dietary supplement and is touted by its manufacturers for use in management of osteoporosis. However, the definitive study performed on more than 400 women with osteoporosis indicated that ipriflavone does not improve bone density or bone turnover, nor does it reduce the occurrence of vertebral fractures.

Moreover, it actually produced a reduction in the number of lymphocytes in a significant number of women, some of whom had not returned to normal two years after stopping the medicine. Therefore, ipriflavone is not recommended and might in fact be dangerous.

NEWER PERSPECTIVES ON NUTRITION AND BONE QUALITY

Dr. Heaney, of Creighton University Medical Center in Omaha, states that as we age we tend to experience more structural loss in our 206 bones beginning at the age of 34. This loss of bone mass expresses the quantity of bone loss. If we eat a smart bone-building diet and supplement with a bone-building team of additional nutrients, we can improve bone strength immediately. Dr. Heaney states that, "Bone-building nutrients add qualitative strength to build and maintain bone strength, independent of the quantity of bone."

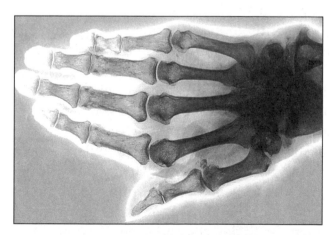

Figure 8.2: The Complexity of Bone and Joint Structure Enables Us to Have Fluid Biomechanical Movements

Far from slowly powering out and down, bone as it ages begins bringing new support systems on line and cross-indexing existing ones in ways it never did before if we daily consume the broad spectrum of bone-building nutrients. Essentially, bone spends decades upgrading itself from a dial-up Internet to a high-speed version, maybe not fully completing the job until midlife, age 45 or so.

> Researchers are coming to the conclusion that midlife—a period increasingly defined as the years from 35 to 65 and even beyond—is a much more creative period for bone-building strength than anyone ever realized.

BE CAREFUL OF FLUORIDE

The word "poison" on your toothpaste tube is now required by U.S. drug regulators who deny the safety of fluoride, particularly for children. Canada only mandates labels that warn consumers not to let small children eat more than a pea-sized amount daily.

Only slightly less poisonous than arsenic, fluoride is worse than lead but is permitted in toothpaste and in Canadian drinking water. City water often has one part per million—100 times the safety level for lead.

At least half the fluoride we consume fuses permanently with bones and teeth, weakening overall health. Skeletal fluorosis is a widespread problem where high levels naturally occur, as in parts of China, India, and Turkey. Apart from bones becoming extremely weak and brittle, fluoride causes premature aging and death, miscarriage, birth defects, and other serious illness.

The vast majority of fluoride we use is a toxic by-product of the super-phosphate fertilizer industry, according to University of Toronto dentistry professor Dr. Hardy Limeback. He says children under three should never have fluoridated toothpaste or tap water, especially in baby formula; developing bones and teeth are particularly vulnerable. He's concerned that most of the children he treats in his Mississauga practice suffer dental fluorosis (porous and easily stained teeth) from tap water, ready-made beverages, and toothpaste.

Limeback's studies show residents of Toronto, which has had fluoridated water for 40 years, have twice the fluoride levels in their hip bones as do those in Montreal, where citizens won the right not to fluoridate in the 1980s. Vancouver has never fluoridated and has a lower cavity rate. Many Canadian municipalities have opted not to fluoridate. Toronto has recently reduced levels from one to .08 parts per million (still 80 times the lead safety level).

Many brands of health food store toothpaste do not contain fluoride.

ADAPTABILITY: IT'S ON OUR SIDE

Surprise! The *Journal of Morphology* published in September 2002 some very interesting and exciting research. Researchers from the University of Jena, in Jena, Germany—as well as researchers from the University of Cape Town, South Africa—examined the microstructure pattern of bone growth in dinosaurs' bone fossil. The conclusion for several species of dinosaurs is that bone-building rates conform exactly to environmental conditions. In years of plentiful nutrients, the dinosaurs' bones grew strong and flexible. In years of low nutrient intake, the bones lost their strength and became weakened.

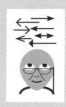 As we age, the brain's hemispheres work in tandem, integrating thought processes more effectively. Maybe our bones are also capable of adapting to better nutrition and become more effective as we age.

This is the basis of *adaptability*. All humans have inherited adaptability hardwired into their brains. Our great, great, great-grandparents survived because they became adaptable. We are the descendants of those who survived because of their adaptability to the environment. Those who did not adapt perished, and their genes went the way of extinction.

Organic chemistry, physiology, biology, and quantum mechanics may come to a universal agreement that bones do not grow denser after midlife, but you are able to more effectively use what you already have, and keep it strong.

Indeed, until quite recently most researchers believed the human brain also followed a fairly predictable developmental arc. It started out arching upwards, gained shape and intellectual strength as it matured, and reached its peak of power and nimbleness by age 40. After that, the brain began a slow decline, clouding up little by little by little until, by age 65 or 70, it had lost much of its ability to retain new information and was fumbling with what it had.

In fact, psychologists are now unanimously agreeing that in midlife, or even later life, for many people the aging process not only does not batter the brain, it actually makes it better. "In midlife," says UCLA neurologist George Bartzokis, "you're beginning to maximize the ability to use the entirety of the information in your brain on an everyday, ongoing, second-to-second basis. Biologically speaking, that's what wisdom is."

As it turns out, most medical researchers bought into the old theory of mental decline until as late as 2003, when the entire framework of their assumptions was proven to be incorrect. Contrary to the focus of past bone research, ultra-fascinating, fast-paced modern research is now suggesting that our 206 bones and 143 joints can grow and get stronger, even in midlife, and well beyond! The head-turning, breakthrough research presented in this book reveals how to keep your bones, structure, posture, and fluid biomechanical movement at peak performance for an entire lifetime.

Another U.N. Issue Regarding Our Diet and Bones

Canadians and Americans are addicted to "cheap, acidifying processed food." The U.N. states that we North Americans spend only 9.7 percent of our income on food, a much smaller share than any other nation. Is it a coincidence we spend a larger percentage (a full 16 percent) on health care than any other nation? The higher the quality of the food you eat, the more nutritious it is and the less of it you'll need to feel satisfied and healthy—with strong nails, teeth, and bones for a lifetime!

CHAPTER 9

Ramp Up Bone-Building Metabolic Exercise

Decades before Tony Little felt the burn and Suzanne Somers thinned her thighs and Oprah Winfrey slimmed down, my grandmother was teaching people how to stay trim and have strong bones, nails, and teeth.

Back in the 1930s, as Nana Marie was getting started, her straight talk on nutrition and fitness was positively revolutionary.

In 1935, when meat and potatoes were a meal and physical fitness was a subculture, Nana Marie opened a combination juice bar and health-food store in Los Angeles. She was affectionately nicknamed, "Herbs, Nuts, Twigs, and Seeds."

Nana Marie promoted daily exercise rather than girdles to keep women trim. She also tried to get people to think positively by peppering her instructions with cheery aphorisms like, "You want a 2010 brain but you're settling for a model-T body."

As fitness and health moved into the mainstream, Nana Marie's star began to fade a little. In the 1980s and 1990s a new generation of glitzy instructors on infomercials promised dramatic results fast, and Nana, who focused on her trademark fundamentals, lost prominence to hawking high-powered gadgets and infomercial staples.

The aerobics revolution of the 1980s and 1990s added theory to the practice of vigorous exercise. To benefit from working, exercise physiologists told us, you had to push your heart rate to 70–85 percent of its maximum, keep pouring out sweat for 30–60 minutes at a crack, and do it all over again five to seven days a week. And researchers kept cranking out fancy data that seemed to confirm what our high school phys ed. teachers shouted: no pain, no gain.

MODERATE EXERCISE

Unfortunately, the aerobics doctrine inspired a few but discouraged too many. However, as it turns out, perspiration isn't the only answer. You can reap enormous health benefits and strong bones with no-sweat exercise— as long as you know what to do. In fact, everything that gets you moving—from gardening, hiking, walking, washing the car, Tai Chi, hatha yoga, Pilates, dancing, aerobics, and stair climbing—can and will contribute to your superior bone health.

"Moderate exercise" is credited in recent research with 18–84 percent reduction of heart disease, 18–50 percent reduction in the overall mortality rate, and a 60 percent increase in bone mineral density (BMD).

I know you're saying that "moderate exercise" must have some catch to it, but it doesn't. A few examples: In the Netherlands, those who walked or biked for at least one hour a week enjoyed a 29 percent lower mortality rate than sedentary people; in North America, research shows walking at least a mile a day reduced the risk of heart disease by 82 percent over a 10-year period; in a Seattle study, gardening for just two hours a week appeared to lower the risk of sudden cardiac death by 66 percent.

You do not have to do your sweat-free exercise all at once. A study of young college students found that daily exercise was equally beneficial whether it occurred in a single 30-minute session, or two 15-minute sessions. The benefits were substantial: in just 12 weeks the students shed nearly 10 lbs each. Medical researchers in England reported similar results, finding that three 10-minute walks a day had the same good effects on lowering cholesterol and stress, while increasing bone mineral density, as a 30-minute daily walk.

Moderate daily exercise can also help reduce hypertension, diabetes, and osteoporosis. It's an essential partner with a good diet for people who need to lose weight or build strong bones. In May 2005, *The Journal of the American Medical Association* published research stating that no-sweat exercise can help reduce and reverse type 2 diabetes by 15–45 percent, dementia by 25–50 percent, breast cancer by 20–30 percent, colon cancer by 30–50 percent, and osteoporosis fractures by a huge 50 percent.

Surprisingly, exercise increases the production of brain-derived neurotrophic factor (BDNF), a chemical that helps brain and bone cells multiply and form new connections. This bigger "circuit board" in the brain or bones means better bone-building and brainpower for life. In February 2006, the journal *Neurology* reported that those who engaged in regular exercise lowered their risk for Parkinson's disease by 60 percent. Dr. William Evans and Dr. Irwin Rosenberg from Tufts University documented that regular exercise reduced the risk of osteoporosis by 62 percent.

WHY THIS SEISMIC SHIFT TO NO-SWEAT EXERCISE?

Human biology and physiology has not changed since Nana Marie began in 1935, but science certainly has. The aerobics doctrine of the 1980s and 1990s is based on experiments that measure how exercise affects aerobic fitness, on how much oxygen your body can absorb (called VO_2 Max) while you're going all out on a treadmill. It is still true that for superior and maximal fitness you have to work out aerobically. But in our fast-paced modern life, don't put an artificial barrier between "exercise" and "physical activity." The intensity of the 1990s aerobic approach has its rewards, but what actually matters most is that you simply get moving.

Harvey B. Simon, M.D., Associate Professor of Medicine at Harvard Medical School, in his new book, *The No Sweat Exercise Plan: Lose Weight, Get Healthy, and Live Longer*, has coined the term "cardiometabolic exercise" (CME) to emphasize the many health benefits of everything from moderate activity, to hitting the elliptical machine, to housework, to washing the car, to walking the dog, to aerobic training. The accompanying graphic assigns Dr. Simon's CME points to selective daily and recreational activities. For general health and gradual weight loss, he wants you to aim for 150 points a day or about 1,000 points a week; for faster weight loss and for healthy bone-repair or bone-building, ramp up to 300 points a day and 2,000 a week.

You get extra benefit by adding exercises for strength, flexibility, core strength, walking, and balance—not at a gym, but at home. Small changes add up quickly!

Learning these techniques is very helpful, not only because they help produce a trim healthy body, but because they can turn ordinary activities into meaningful exercise.

Little Things Mean a Lot

The value of an activity depends on the physical exertion involved. Pick a daily target score (150 points is moderate) and then track your progress.

Cardiometabolic-exercise (CME) points for selected activities (all activities last 30 minutes, except sleep [8 hours] and stair climbing [10 minutes]):

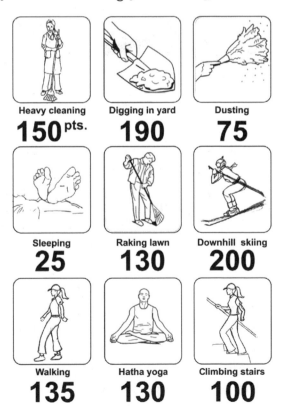

Heavy cleaning	Digging in yard	Dusting
150pts.	**190**	**75**
Sleeping	Raking lawn	Downhill skiing
25	**130**	**200**
Walking	Hatha yoga	Climbing stairs
135	**130**	**100**

CORE STRENGTH

Millions of aerobic-minded boomers are discovering that a strong torso, though hard-earned, is absolutely essential for long-term fitness. For decades we promoted aerobic exercise as critical for cardiovascular health, and the importance of regular weight training for maintaining muscle mass in the arms and legs.

But, since 2004, physical therapists and personal coaches have begun urging people, especially middle-aged sedentary people, to keep their core muscles strong and supple in order to maintain and improve balance, posture, mobility, and bone health. Recent studies prove that people with strong muscles in their abdomen, buttocks, and pelvis get fewer fractures and have both better posture and better balance.

Optimally, when the legs, arms, and neck move, the core muscles in the abdomen keep the body stable. Dr. John Berardi, Assistant Professor at the University of Texas, President of Science Link, Inc., and an exercise physiology master who works with prominent Olympic athletes, says, "Think of your two arms, two legs, and neck as spokes on a wheel and your core is the center. If the core is weak or unbalanced, your body will be off balance and less effective during both daily activities and exercise." He continues, "Therefore, core conditioning isn't as straightforward as pumping a barbell. You need to isolate, balance, and strengthen your core muscles in addition to using a strength training routine that is customized for your body type." Personnel at your local gym or exercise facility can quickly help you determine your body type and develop an effective core-strengthening program specific for you.

The Results Are in

Core strength training can help you keep up your pace for the rest of your life.

The results are in: Core training, along with cardio exercise and working out with weights, keeps your balance, posture, and bone health at an optimum for longer. Core workouts, although not always easy to begin with, are actually fun! Here are five core exercises to tighten up your midsection and build strong bones.

Pilates:

Once a dancer's secret, the decades-old core builder is now mainstream. In 2005, 12 million people in North America tried Pilates, which is based on the techniques of Joseph Pilates, who trained dancers, actors, and athletes in his New York studio.

Tai Chi and Qigong:

These ancient Eastern techniques, which originated in China, are done in slow, rhythmic motion with deep concentration and smooth breathing. They have quickly gained Western converts. The focus is on balance, gracious but powerful motion, breathing, and a flexible, strong trunk.

Qigong is a therapeutic Chinese practice that has been used for thousands of years to cultivate, restore, and balance vital body energy or *qi*.

Yoga:

An ancient system originating in India of deep concentration, fluid movements, flexibility, breathing, and core strength has been "rekindled" by no-nonsense author and teacher B.K.S. Iyengar of India, now 87, and by various yoga magazines and thousands of yoga instructors in every community.

Rebounding:

Rebound exercise is done on a small trampoline. It strengthens every cell in the body at the same time. As you bounce, you accelerate and decelerate on the same plane, or vertically, with gravity. In normal exercise you oppose gravity with just one force.

The cells of the body, especially the lymphatic and core muscles, know how to adjust to an increased force of gravity. They respond by getting stronger with better balance and posture.

Exercise Ball:

The decade-old exercise ball is also mainstream now. Exercise balls come in various sizes and are an excellent way to develop balance, symmetry of all core muscles, and good posture. Simply sitting on a ball and bouncing straight up and down with controlled balance, rhythmic breathing, and flow strengthens core muscles.

THE BREAKTHROUGH BONE-BUILDER EXERCISE PROGRAM

After years of research I have combined the benefits of Pilates, yoga, Tai Chi, Qigong, rebounding, and the exercise ball into either a 30- or 60-minute home workout. Of course, it would be of great benefit for you to join classes in your area in any of these six core-building exercises, designed to give you great bone health, balance, posture, and core strength.

You may consider purchasing the following:

- a pair of 2 lb ankle weights $ 15.00
- a pair of both 10 and 20 lb barbells   50.00
- an exercise ball   30.00
- a soft bounce rebounder such as a   250.00
  Needak®

Total Expenditures $345.00

The Beginner

Follow the sequence of the next 12 bone-building no-sweat exercises. To begin with, rotate from one to 12 in order, spending just one minute on each. After one week, do this 12-minute routine twice a day, then three times a day.

The Intermediary

Once you have the routine down pat, increase each no-sweat exercise to two-and-a-half minutes once a day and build up to three times a day.

The Master

Do the routine of no-sweat exercises for five minutes each once a day and build up to two times a day. Be very conscious of maintaining good posture, rhythmic breathing, and balance at all times. Start to feel the "burn" in core muscles and visualize all 206 of your bones becoming stronger and healthier.

DO NOT UNDERESTIMATE THIS BREAKTHROUGH BONE-BUILDER EXERCISE PROGRAM

A recent study measured bone mineral density (BMD) among women ages 50–60 who had practiced Tai Chi daily for over four years. They were compared with the same number of women, with the same average age of 55, who did not practice Tai Chi. The BMD in weight-bearing bones among the women doing daily Tai Chi was almost 15 percent higher than in the non-Tai Chi group. This study was reported in the *Archives of Physical Medical Rehabilitation* in 2002.

Another very interesting study measured physical outcomes in girls trained in yoga compared to non-practising girls. The *Indian Journal of Physiology and Pharmacology* in 1997 reported the girls doing daily ha-tha yoga exercises had improved reaction time, balance, coordination, muscle power, motor skills, respiratory endurance, and visual perception.

The American College of Traditional Chinese Medicine in San Francisco, California, measured the electrical conductivity (energy flow) in 24 acupuncture points, with 29 participants doing a two-day workshop on Qigong. By the end of the second day, there was better overall balance of energy (*qi*) between the various acupuncture points in 100 percent of all the 29 test subjects.

Teens

Teens are especially at risk for poor bone development because their bones are growing so rapidly. Boys and girls from ages nine to 18 need 1,300 mg of calcium each day, more than any other age group. Parents can help teens by making sure they eat four servings of calcium-rich and vitamin D3-fortified foods a day. At least one hour a day of physical activities—like running, skateboarding, sports, and dance—is also critical. Studies show that only half of all teens exercise vigorously on a regular basis, and one-fourth do not exercise at all. But take note: Extreme physical exercise, when combined with undereating, can weaken teens' bones. In young women this situation can lead to a damaging lack of menstrual periods. Teens who miss adding bone to their skeletons during these critical years might never make it up.

RIGHT AND LEFT SIDE BODY EQUILIBRIUM AND ADAPTATION

All too often, we forget that weight-resistance training (dumbbells, barbells, weight machines) is not the only form of resistance training for weight control, lean muscle tissue, and strong, healthy bones. Resistance training is a process of overloading your muscular system so the body can *adapt* with increased flexibility, balance, strength, endurance, and sheer power. Newer forms of resistance training utilize body weight in motion, exercise balls, rebounders, Tai Chi, Pilates, hatha yoga, and unstable surfaces.

Initially, there will be a difference in terms of balance, strength, coordination, and endurance between your right and left sides. One side is dominant and we unconsciously favor it. Our bodies tend to be "out of balance" left to right and front to back. This is the result of being right-handed or left-handed in the variety of activities we perform on a daily basis including:

1. eating

2. writing

3. drinking

4. gardening

5. opening doors

6. preparing food

7. carrying groceries

8. doing routine home cleaning and driving

9. exercising; playing golf, tennis, soccer, basketball; dancing, etc.

10. using a cell phone, land phone, computer, BlackBerry, etc.

In general, a body that favors the right side or left side is out of balance at ground zero, in your core muscles, and does not operate as efficiently as a body in balance. Researchers refer to this balance as *physiological homeostasis* or *equilibrium*. We are all preprogrammed for either a right-side or left-side dominance, termed "the malalignment syndrome."

The following 12 exercises will automatically put your body back into balance so you will move better, play better, feel better, and allow your body to adapt to an equilibrium resulting in better bones. Do all core exercises slowly, paying close attention to your core muscles as you move and breathe deeply, exhaling as you exert and flex your muscles, inhaling as you return to the starting position.

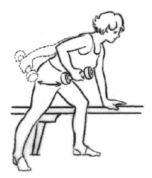

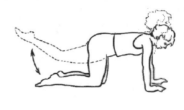

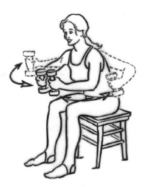

Exercise 1

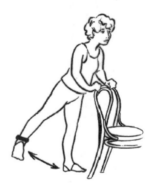

Exercise 2

Exercise 3

Exercise 4

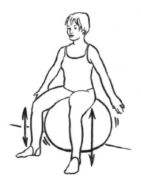

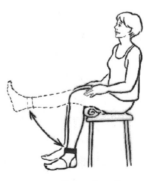

Exercise 5

Exercise 6

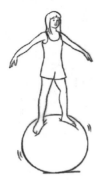

Exercise 7

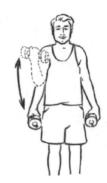

Exercise 8

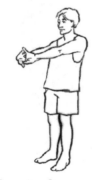

Exercise 9

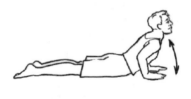

Exercise 10

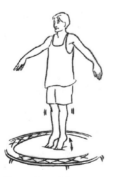

Exercise 11

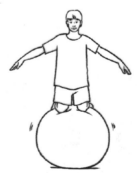

Exercise 12

BETTER EXERCISES, BETTER HEALTH, BETTER BONES

As North Americans, we are living a vast, unsupervised experiment. Never before has any nation been so physically inactive; spent so much time indoors under artificial lights passively watching television, video movies, DVDs, playing video games, reading newspapers, or listening to our iPods; eaten so much processed foods; drunk so many artificial pops and juices; taken so many drugs and medications; exposed ourselves to so much electromagnetic radiation, household chemical "off-gassing" or informational pollution; experienced such pervasive and acute stress or anxiety; and undergone so many necessary or elective surgical procedures. We also consume alcohol and recreational drugs at an alarming, accelerated rate.

Dietary excesses and deficiencies, lifestyle factors, smoking, toxic metals, prescription or recreation drug dependency, alcohol, stress or anxiety, and physical inactivity have combined to make weak bones, poor teeth, and brittle nails the "silent epidemic" of the current decade from 2000 to 2010.

In a large-scale study of Harvard University alumni, those who participated in exercise activities of moderate intensity had a 23–29 percent lower risk of dying from any cause compared to the participants who never participated in exercise. In discussing these findings, the principal author of the study, Dr. Paffenbarger, suggests that, "Each hour of moderate physical activity brings one, two or even three extra hours of healthy life," as reported in the *Berkeley Wellness Newsletter*.

Exercise builds and maintains bone at all ages. It is absolutely essential for optimum bone development in the young, and without exercise the aging bone is limited in its ability to regenerate. Nutrition alone cannot support maximum peak bone mass or maintain optimum bone health as you age.

Exercise is not optional—it is mandatory! All children and adults should engage in regular and vigorous exercise outdoors. Keep physically active all day long.

A LITTLE EXERCISE CAN DRAMATICALLY IMPROVE BONE-BUILDING

Aerobic and Anaerobic Exercise

The physiological benefits of exercise are improved:

- bone-repair and bone-building functions
- overall muscle coordination and strength
- brain and neurotransmitter functions
- oxygenation of all 100 trillion cells
- overall stress reduction
- long-term weight loss
- memory and mood
- bowel function
- cardio fitness
- independence
- posture
- sleep

There are three components of proper exercise:

1. Stretching
   - reduces potential injuries while improving flexibility and balance
2. Aerobic exercise
   - increases lung capacity and heart rate
   - lowers glucose, insulin, and cortisol levels
   - raises "feel good" levels of the hormones serotonin and endorphins
3. Anaerobic exercise
   - releases bone-building and anti-aging growth hormone (HGH), insulin-like growth factor (IGF-1), and testosterone

The beneficial drop in blood glucose and insulin levels is accompanied by an increase in HGH and testosterone in both men and women who exercise. In men and women alike, the effect is an increase in bone mineral density (BMD) and muscle strength.

In women, these effects are moderated by the hormones estrogen and progesterone, so bone-building resistance training doesn't produce hair growth or bulging muscles.

Strength training can be just as effective for older people as younger people.

Bone-Building Walking

Walking, cycling, aerobics, water aerobics, swimming, dancing, jogging, a treadmill, gardening, an elliptical machine, or callisthenics are all good bone-building aerobic exercises.

I want to emphasize that walking allows you to maintain a strong core while maximizing large and small muscle groups, as well as concentrating on rhythmic breathing. Walking keeps the neck and shoulders relaxed while working the lower and upper arms, your gluts, and the lower and upper legs.

Begin a walking program slowly with a maximum of 20 minutes a day. As you become more proficient, every seven days you will be able to walk further and faster until you reach a 45-minute power-walk pace.

A long-term walking program, outside in the fresh air with natural sunlight, elevates several beneficial hormone levels, builds bone, burns fat, reduces acute stress, and lowers food intake because your body switches to burning stored body fat for fuel instead of glucose. Many towns and cities have beautiful urban parks to walk in. Consider a 20-minute walk during your lunch hour and organize others to join you for a power walk.

Simple Walking Is a Good Aerobic Exercise

Always inhale deeply through your nose, consciously pulling air deep into your lungs. Imagine the air rushing into your core, energizing your core with strength and a vital life force. Exhale slowly through your mouth with your lips slightly open.

Most people walk to burn calories, loosen their tense muscles, lubricate joints, and for cardio training. You can have all of these benefits plus complementary bone-building.

Once you can walk faster and farther, the extended lateral movement of your arms and legs is an excellent way to develop a lean, trim midsection and tight buttocks. Try walking in a park, beside the bank of a river, or a place where you won't be interrupted by traffic.

Walking, cycling, jogging, tennis, racquetball, stair stepping, using a stationary bike or elliptical machine, and swimming are aerobic exercises that increase breathing, heart rate, circulation, weight loss, and benefit bone-building. While walking, you prime your muscles and prepare your cardiovascular and respiratory systems for increased activity.

During the first 20 minutes of walking, your body shifts from burning glucose to burning glycogen, stored energy in your liver and muscles. As this happens, your body begins releasing human growth hormone (HGH) and decreases bloodstream glucose and insulin levels.

After 20 minutes, glycogen stores become depleted and fat becomes your primary fuel. From 20–40 minutes, testosterone levels start to rise. After 45 minutes of walking, cycling, jogging, or swimming both testosterone and HGH levels begin to decline. Therefore, after 45 minutes of aerobic exercise, it is an ideal time to do 15–30 minutes of weight-resistance training before HGH and testosterone levels decline any further.

Aerobic exercise promotes body coordination and critical oxygen exchange. These exercises can improve insulin sensitivity and increase *erythropoietin*, which is the hormone that boosts red blood cell formation. Finally, aerobic exercise reduces the cortisol stress hormone levels by triggering the body's natural relaxation response.

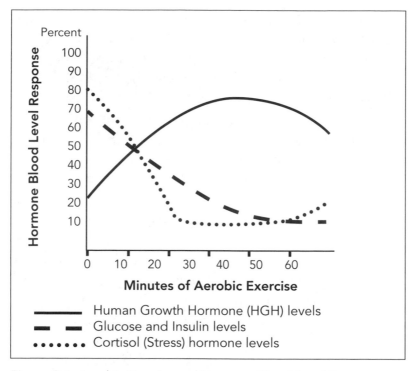

Figure 9.1: Aerobic Exercise and Hormone Blood Level Response

The body is a highly adaptive piece of machinery and adaptation is what it does best! When the body is repeatedly presented with the same challenge, it will adapt, allowing it to meet the challenge with less effort. Because of the body's adaptive response, aerobic exercise, such as long-distance running or biking, longer than 45 minutes is counterproductive. Instead of burning more calories, the body adapts, and becomes more efficient and in fact burns fewer calories. It is, therefore, much more productive to begin weight training after 45 minutes of cardiovascular exercise than to continue working your body aerobically.

The following graph demonstrates the hormonal benefits of weight-resistance training for 30 minutes after 45 minutes of aerobic exercise.

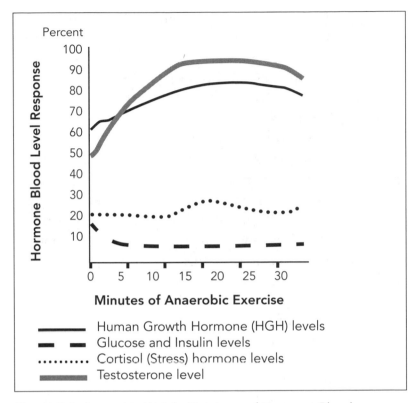

Figure 9.2: Anaerobic Weight Training and Hormone Blood Level Response

Interval Training

Interval training is a smart way to work around the body's adaptive response to sustained exercise like walking, running, biking, swimming, spinning, or working out on a treadmill or elliptical machine or stair stepper or stationary bike. Instead of maintaining a steady pace for the entire distance of time of exercise, build some extra exertion (sprint) and recovery intervals. Surprisingly, you build stronger muscles and stronger, more resilient heart and lungs.

The technique is simple. For your 45 minutes of aerobics do: (1) a two-minute faster pace or sprint speed at about 80–90 percent of your maximum possible exertion; (2) then back off the pace for five minutes at 50 percent maximum possible exertion. Simply repeat this cycle for 45 minutes. Interval training also reduces the risk of exercise-induced injuries.

People who perform aerobic and anaerobic exercises three to five times a week perform better, feel better, and think better, regardless of their age. All exercise releases "feel good" neurotransmitters like serotonin, and pain-killing beta endorphins. The additional benefits are that exercise reduces insulin levels and reduces the stress hormone cortisol. And there's always the extra bonus of stronger, more flexible bones and muscles, and improved body image.

Although it may be trendy to say you work out, it is not possible or necessary for everyone to have an abdominal six-pack or washboard abs. You need to exercise smarter and think of exercise in a new way. We need to realize that exercising smarter means building muscle and bone strength, balance, and a better range of motion through a wide variety of exercises. Our lack of exercise is killing us!

MEASURE FOR METABOLIC HEALTH: DO YOU MEASURE UP?

The body mass index (BMI), a popular formula that combines height and weight, has a flaw in it. Fit people with dense muscle mass consistently register as overweight and unhealthy.

Dr. Jean-Pierre Despres, of Laval University in Quebec City, has championed another measure for metabolic health: waist circumference. In a series of recent studies, researchers found that a larger waist circumference is a good indicator for metabolic syndrome, a constellation of physiological changes that can lead to diabetes, heart disease, reduced bone-building, and osteoporosis.

Dr. Despres says of the simple measure, "I call it a vital sign." It's a kind of wake-up call or early warning system, since reducing expanding waistlines cuts the risk of heart disease and osteoporosis. Ideal waistline measurements for men are under 40 inches and for women under 30 inches.

The ideal percentage of body fat is 12–20 percent for men, and 18–26 percent for women. But it's not healthy to be significantly above or below this percentage, and I recommend staying on the lean side of these ranges.

BREATHE DEEPLY SO OXYGEN CAN NEUTRALIZE THE ACIDS

When you exercise you create an abundance of a volatile liquid acid called carbonic acid (H_2CO_3). When you breathe deeply and rhythmically while exercising, the extra oxygen quickly kicks in to downregulate and separate carbonic acid into carbon dioxide (CO_2) and water (H_2O). You exhale the carbon dioxide out through your lungs and pass the water out through perspiration and urine. Deep breathing will increase your lung capacity (VO_2 Max) and increase microcirculation of alkalinizing oxygen to cells in all your bones and extremities.

Remember to stretch before and after you exercise to maintain your full range of motion in major joints. Combining rhythmic breathing and stretching helps to remove increased acids due to exercise, and stretching primes your body for further exercise. It is also a good technique to use throughout the day for improving balance between spontaneous, acidifying active reactions (the automatic-pilot sympathetic nervous system) and more conscious, alkaline, and calming reactions to daily life (which is the parasympathetic nervous system).

THE GOOD AND BAD OF SUNLIGHT EXPOSURE DURING EXERCISE

You must be both wise and careful because sunlight contains very high-intensity, high-energy ultraviolet rays called UVA and UVB. The sun's rays can penetrate the outer epidermal layers of skin and damage cellular genes in the basal skin layer. These are living skin cells that are rapidly dividing and differentiating into various cellular networks of external skin. Melanoma, the most serious kind of skin cancer, is ignited by excessive UVA and UVB sunrays in these basal skin cells.

Xanthophyll carotenoids (a family of phytonutrients) do not convert to vitamin A like beta-carotene does. This carotenoid family is made up of astaxanthin, canthaxantin, lutein, and zeaxanthin found primarily in huge bioavailable abundance in egg yolks. They are very protective, in your skin, against ultraviolet A (UVA) and ultraviolet B (UVB) sunray radiation. Furthermore, they protect your eyes from macular degeneration and support bone-building.

We humans have evolved with a protective skin pigment called melanin that literally absorbs UVA and UVB wavelengths and turns the skin brown. When walking in full sunlight, try to walk in the early morning or evening, and never between 10 a.m. and 3 p.m. You require only

15 minutes of early morning or late afternoon sun on your unprotected hands, arms, and face to produce sufficient vitamin D3 for enhanced bone-building.

The best safeguards are to wear protective clothing, sunscreen, a hat, use a supplemental softgel containing 2–4 mg of astaxanthin, and eat organic, vegetable-fed, free-range chicken eggs. Be sure that your sunscreen is natural and hypoallergenic containing titanium dioxide and zinc oxide for a high refractive index with no harmful chemicals. Your sunscreen must state on the label that it protects against both ultraviolet A (UVA) and ultraviolet B sunray radiation (95% don't). It should include vitamin E, aloe vera, borage oil, and green tea extract to prevent skin irritations. Your local natural food store will carry such a sunscreen.

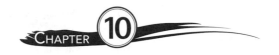

Chapter 10

Five Bone-Building Tips for Every Decade of Your Life: Do a Menu Makeover

AN AWESOME BIOLOGICAL JOLT

Genetically we have evolved, but so have the ever-available processed, synthetic, refined foods. Can they fuel our magnificent 100 trillion cells? Today, genetics and lifestyle are colliding. To have your bone-building vitality, and brainpower operating at optimum, it is critical to fuel yourself with a food selection true to your ancient genetic origin and makeup.

Our shift from hunting and gathering to agriculture, and from the Industrial Revolution to our present electronic computer age, has drastically changed human nutrition with an extremely detrimental biological jolt, which in turn has promoted heart disease, cancer, stroke, depression, diabetes, osteoporosis, and a prevailing sense of drop-dead fatigue.

Change the environment knowingly or unknowingly and the environment is guaranteed to change you. "Food-stuff"—the degraded foods of modern commerce—are unfamiliar to your genes, brain, and bones, triggering serious intracellular communication breakdowns and leading to daily bone deterioration.

There is now a worrisome decrease in our consumption of lean, high-quality protein; very low-density complex carbohydrates, such as vegetables, greens, salads, spices, and herbs; and moderate-density complex carbohydrates, such as fruit, berries, and minimally processed grains. These "cell-friendly" foods contain a little naturally occurring sugar for a steady energy supply and a lot of life-supportive fiber, water, vitamins, minerals, trace minerals, antioxidants, and bone-building phytonutrients.

Knowledge is power when it comes to a lifetime of superior health!

BONE-BUILDING TIPS FOR CHILDREN, TEENS, AND ADULTS TO BOOST BONES TO THE MAX

No matter how impeccable you think your diet is, there are always ways to take it to the next level. All it takes is a few easy inclusions. These five simple dietary inclusions will bring you maximum bone-building and the healthiest, happiest you. The research evidence is so compelling that if you add the following five bone-building tips to your family's daily diet, you will keep their metabolic harmony and bones functioning at peak levels for a lifetime.

Bon appétit!

Jump Start Your Day with a One-Minute Protein Power Shake

Start the day right by having a protein power shake for breakfast to feel full until noon, reduce cravings, lower cholesterol levels, dramatically increase vitamin and mineral absorption, create energy galore, and keep your teeth brilliant and bones strong.

Furthermore, the *Journal of Nutrition*, in June 2004, and the *American Journal of Clinical Nutrition*, in June 2000, printed solid scientific research that suggested using high-alpha, 100 percent whey isolate protein powder made with a low-temperature cross-flow, micro-filtration technique. This produces a whey isolate that is greater than 90 percent protein, and more than 99 percent undenatured. High-alpha whey protein powder can turn "on" internal survival switches that:

1. give you a staggering decrease in body fat

2. give you an increase in lean muscle mass

3. raise the "good mood" levels of the hormone serotonin, reducing depression, anxiety, and indecisiveness

4. lower cortisol (stress) bloodstream concentrations, thus improving relaxation, memory, and a general sense of well-being

5. reduce hunger, food cravings, and food intake between meals by raising the appetite-busting hormones leptin and ghrelin; and the "I'm full" hormones cholecystokinin (CCK); and glucagon-like peptide-1 (GLP-1); and downregulating the endocannabinoid system, a network of receptor cells in the brain, the liver, and fat tissue that regulates hunger by linking appetite to the body's reward and satisfaction system

6. accelerate both critical mineral and fish oil absorption for superior bone-building.

Start Every Day with a Healthy Breakfast

Let us get one thing established right from the beginning. A great day depends upon a nutritious breakfast and high-octane fuel as healthy food all day long. Start your day with a dynamically balanced protein power shake that I created for gold medal-winning Olympic athletes.

The Ultimate Breakfast Protein Power Shake Recipe

- 8 oz of water, unsweetened rice milk, soy milk, hemp milk, almond milk, or organic skim milk
- 2–4 heaping tbsps of organic, low-fat plain soy or dairy yogurt
- 2 scoops of high-alpha whey protein isolate powder
- 1 full cup of any fresh or frozen berry, such as blueberries, blackberries, or raspberries
- 2 tbsps of both organic flaxseeds and sesame seeds, 30 g each, ground fresh in a coffee grinder for the lignan fibers and the short-chain omega-3 fats
- ½ tsp of organic borage oil for the bioactive omega-6 fatty acid gamma linolenic acid, or simply swallow one 500 mg capsule of evening primrose oil for biologically active omega-6 fatty acids

Blend all ingredients in a blender for 10 seconds on low so that you do not denature the whey protein isolate powder. Tip: Add the high-alpha whey protein powder last.

- 1 softgel of enteric-coated ultrapure fish oils allowing 300 percent better absorption and no fishy aftertaste; or use 1 tbsp of liquid oil. Use fish oils rich in EPA and DHA super-critical fats that your brain needs daily for good moods, enhanced memory, and increased brainpower—and your bones need for maximum bone-building and strength.

Note: Always take your enteric-coated fish oil capsules or liquid with your breakfast protein power shake. The fish oil gets dispersed in the preformed emulsions from the high-alpha whey isolate protein powder. These fat emulsions are an ideal delivery system to maximize fish oil absorption.

High-alpha whey protein isolate powder is alkalinizing!

Choose the Right Color-Coded Fruit, Berries, and Vegetables

In the December 2004 edition of the *Journal of the American College of Nutrition*, researchers from the University of Texas discovered that many fruits and vegetables today, because of selective breeding and genetic modification, are larger but have less taste and nutrients. They are also picked green so that they can ship better.

Big red flavorless strawberries, and tasteless and overly hard tomatoes are the result of selective breeding by commercial growers who want more pith and water (pith is the fibrous part of fruits and vegetables) for produce to ship well, look good, and weigh more, but they contain less vitamins, minerals, and phytonutrients (disease-fighting compounds in all fruit and vegetables).

It is the polyphenol (a phytonutrient in produce) content of fruit and vegetables that gives them color, taste, and critical bone-building micronutrients aimed at specific molecular targets in osteoblast cells. These micronutrients are needed to activate enzymes involved in important metabolic communication pathways in bone cell-to-cell signaling routes. Furthermore, volumes of scientific evidence prove that polyphenols activate sluggish enzymes in bone-building cells that have become derailed because of suboptimal micronutrient deficiencies over years.

Always choose produce with less interior pulp and more skin surface. For example, choose cherry tomatoes or plum tomatoes over large tomatoes, apricots over peaches, any berry over a large pear, a small apple over a large one, sprouts, broccoli, kale, Swiss chard, herbs, spices, parsley, watercress over large potatoes, turnips, or cauliflower.

It is on the surface of a vegetable, salad, fruit, or berry that the colorful, bone-building, ancient color codes form. Each color is a particular blend of powerful, disease-fighting phytonutrients. Color your plate at every meal by grating color-intense vegetables, herbs, and spices on top of your plate with a stainless steel grater for gourmet visual appeal.

Use Colorful Vegetables Often

Make vegetables a main part of lunch and dinner. Cook extra vegetables at dinner, then use them for snacks or at breakfast or other meals the following day. Creatively look to add vegetables, herbs, and spices to everything you eat.

Plan one or two large or small salads each day. Make a large, colorful salad your main evening meal and add

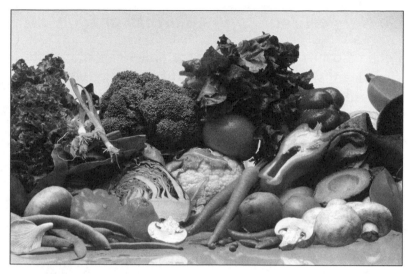

Figure 10.1: Colorful vegetables

steamed vegetables, a small baked yam and a protein serving (beans, chicken, salmon, cottage cheese, tempeh, or firm tofu).

Very little enzyme activity is lost when vegetables are steamed "crunchy tender," and several nutrients are more bioavailable when vegetables are cooked. For example, the red carotenoid lycopene is released when cooking breaks down the cellulose matrix that was trapping it. The important thing is to make sure your vegetables are not overcooked. You can steam them or quickly cook them in a wok with macadamia nut oil, which has proven to be the best cooking oil. Add a handful of fresh herbs, a dash of spices, and you have created an elegant meal.

One helpful tip I often use is to take a cup of raw greens and mix it with something hot so the greens wilt. For example, as a base, put spinach, arugula, or Swiss chard under a piece of chicken breast, fish fillet, a patty of tempeh, lentils, or split peas. In the fall or winter try adding warm wilted greens to your salad.

Do Not Peel Your Apples, Carrots, or Eggplant

Peeling colorful fruit and vegetables can eliminate a significant portion of the colorful polyphenols (phyto-nutrients) because they are in higher concentrations in the outer parts than in the inner parts. The exception is for deep-pigmented fruit like cherries, strawberries, blue-berries, and kiwi, in which they also occur in the flesh.

The polyphenols accumulate in the outer and aerial tissues (skin and leaves) because their biosynthesis is stimulated by sunlight. Major differences in polyphenol concentrations exist between pieces of fruit on the same tree, and even between different sides of a single piece of fruit, depending on the exposure to sunlight.

Similarly, in leafy vegetables such as lettuce, kale, Swiss chard, and cabbage, the polyphenol concentration is 10 times higher in outer leaves than in inner light-colored leaves. This unique phenomenon also accounts for the higher polyphenol and nutrient content of small berries over large fruit and cherry tomatoes to standard tomatoes, because they have better proportions of skin to whole fruit—and more surface area is exposed to sunlight—making more polyphenols.

Are Fruit and Vegetable Waxes Safe?

Have you ever wondered if the glossy wax that is frequently present on cucumbers and apples is safe to eat? Fruit and vegetable waxes are meant to reduce shrinkage from water loss in produce, improve appear-ance by adding a shiny film, and to sometimes provide a carrier for fungicides or other chemical agents to prevent microbial decay, according to the *Journal of Agricultural Food Chemistry*. This same journal lists two common waxing formulas:

1. 18.6 percent oxidized polyethylene, 3.4 percent oleic acid, 2.8 percent morpholine, 0.01 percent polydimethyl-siloxane antifoam in a wax base

2. 9.5 percent shellac, 8.3 percent carnauba wax, 3.3 percent morpholine, 1.7 percent oleic acid, 0.17 percent ammonia, 0.01 percent polydimethyl-siloxane antifoam in a wax base

Fruits and vegetables that are waxed include apples, avocados, bell peppers, cucumbers, grapefruits, lemons, limes, oranges, pineapples, and tomatoes. Since many of these fruits and vegetables are peeled and the peel is not consumed, only a few common fruits and vegetables present a problem since I want you to consume the colorful, nutrient-rich peel. Waxes generally cannot be removed by regular washing.

I prefer my fruit and vegetables wax-free. It is prudent to purchase organic apples, tomatoes, and cucumbers that are not waxed. Local farm produce stands offer fresh produce with no wax. Ask the produce manager at your favorite store to demand more produce from suppliers without wax coatings.

The Ancient Diet Your Brain and Bones Demand

Your bones and brain are organic structures. One hundred percent of the foods you feed to your cells determine their architectural structure, their optimum energy output potential, their ability to function, and your daily rejuvenation potential.

Your body's hardwired bone network communication systems are based on the *available enzymes* found in vegetables, wild greens, nuts, seeds, roots, herbs, spices, fruits, sea vegetables, grass-fed, lean animals, and fish that your ancestors gathered or hunted.

Your biological ancestors instinctively learned to use *naturally protective antioxidants* from freshly gathered plants, such as wild greens, to protect their oxygen-based life processes. Their bodies also learned to use *naturally protective phytonutrients* from freshly gathered plants to protect and restore their cells, bones, vital energy, digestive tracts, organs, and communication networks from daily wear-and-tear, plus eliminate ever-lurking bacteria, viruses, parasites, yeast overgrowth, and carcinogens. Food always has been, and always will be, the best medicine.

Food Source Polyphenols Prevent Rapid Bone Turnover

Volumes of recent, solid, scientific research demonstrates that dietary sources of green salads; color-coded vegetables; in season "cell-friendly" fruits, berries, and melons; "green drinks"; whole organic grains; zingy fermented foods like yogurt or kiefer; and a comprehensive, broad-spectrum micronutrient bone-building supplement contain a class of food-based polyphenols (phytonutrients) that routinely *prevent* bone-breakdown osteoclast cells from becoming aggressively overactive.

Polyphenols increase the electrochemical gradient at the active receptor sites of absorption, embedded in the lipid bilayer, of every bone's cell membrane. These busy absorption receptor sites are called Ca^{2+} (free calcium) channels. The polyphenols are lipophilic (fat soluble) and once in the fatty bone cell membrane, they do three significant and noteworthy functions:

1. Polyphenols create transcription signals that increase the volume and strength of the voltage in Ca^{2+} pumps, which open the "inward gating properties" (absorption sites on cells open to absorb bone-building nutrients) of bone-building cells, increasing calcium concentrations, and successfully transporting calcium and other super-critical bone-building micronutrients into the matrix of new bone tissue development.

2. Polyphenols are extremely powerful antioxidants that are essential for preserving and maintaining cell wall membrane quality, fluidity, and functions, since they are also hydrophilic (water soluble).

3. Polyphenols balance cellular and metabolic regulators that regulate the bidirectional communication pathways between osteoblast (bone-building) and osteoclast (bone-breakdown) cells for healthy bone function and a balanced, homeostatic equilibrium.

Dr. Leticia Rao, Ph.D., and colleagues, demonstrated during *in vitro* studies that it is the active polyphenols in the "green drink" *greens+* that increased and stimulated the inward gating properties of osteoblast cells. A polyphenol's biochemical potential favors boosting bone-building rates and no doubt will also favor decelerating bone-breakdown rates, creating stronger bones at any age, for a lifetime! These results demonstrate, for the first time, that the ancient, color-coded foods containing polyphenol pigments such as those found in *greens+* significantly promote osteoblast bone-building, and suggest that polyphenols play an essential role in regulating healthy bone metabolism and growth—at any age—for a lifetime!

Medicinal Antioxidants That Only Food Provides

The term "antioxidant" applies to many different vitamins, minerals, and food-based chemicals called polyphenols that are responsible for giving fruits and vegetables their color-codes. These compounds serve as antioxidants, but they also have other health-promoting functions. They protect against stroke, heart disease, ADD, ADHD, and common forms of cancer, including breast and prostate. Antioxidants lower inflammation and are powerful inhibitors of bone-breakdown and osteoporosis.

The U.S. Department of Agriculture's (USDA) Human Nutrition Research Center, at Tufts University near Boston, developed a scale—the "oxygen radical absorbency capacity" scale, or ORAC—to rate the antioxidant content of individual foods. The following tables show the fruits and vegetables with the highest ORAC scores.

The USDA scientists found that 10 servings of fruits and vegetables per day provide 3,000–3,500 ORAC points—high-level protection against serious illnesses such as heart disease, stroke, cancer, and osteoporosis. My recommendations give you 5,000 ORAC points daily.

It's important to keep in mind that these and other fruits and vegetables contain substances that have multiple functions, in addition to their antioxidant effects. Broccoli, for example, contains a substance known as sulphoraphane, which has been shown to detoxify tissues and the blood and stimulate the body's cancer-fighting mechanisms. Similar compounds exist in kale, parsley, Swiss chard, collard greens, watercress, other green vegetables, and the "green drink" *greens+*, which supply vitamin K1, which, in turn, converts to vitamin K2 and ignites protein chaperones to guide calcium into bones.

High-ORAC Fruits

Fruit (per cup)	ORAC Score
Blueberries	2,400
Blackberries	2,400
Strawberries	1,540
Raspberries	1,220
Plums	949
Oranges	750
Red grapes	739
Cherries	670
Kiwi fruit	610

High-ORAC Vegetables

Vegetable (per cup)	ORAC Score
Swiss chard	1,800
Kale	1,770
Spinach	1,260
Bean sprouts	980
Brussels sprouts	980
Alfalfa sprouts	930
Broccoli flowerets	890
Beets	840
Red bell peppers	710

The Ancient Rules of Color-Coded Eating

Studies about individual foods, vitamins, phytonutrients, antioxidants, and minerals sometimes conflict. But
scientists are very clear on the 10 foods you need to eat
daily to boost your bone-building health to the maximum. Follow the Rules of Color-Coded Eating by using
a rainbow of bright colors in your vegetable and salad
selections to color your plate at every meal.

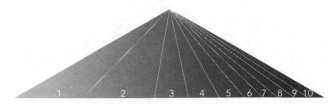

Figure 10.2: The Ancient Rules of Color-Coded Eating

1. **Water:** Eight full glasses a day with a squeeze of lemon or lime juice, 2 cups of herbal tea

2. **Color-Coded Vegetables:** Vary the seasonal colors and textures, 4 or more cups a day

3. **Color-Coded Fruit and Berries:** Vary the bright colors by season, 2 cups a day

4. **Animal- and/or Plant-Based Protein:** Eat lean protein at each of your three meals; children 15 gm a meal; teenagers 20 gm; women 20–25 gm; men 30–35 gm at each meal

5. **Whole Grains:** Brown rice, whole wheat, amaranth, spelt, 1 cup a day; and/or

   Starchy Vegetables: Yams, sweet potatoes, squash, turnips, 1 cup a day

6. **Good Fats:** Extra-virgin olive oil, 2 tbsps a day; cook with macadamia nut oil; try coconut oil instead of butter; use EPA- and "bone-smart" DHA-rich fish oils; use borage or evening primrose oil—combine the best of these fats by daily using an omega-3, -6, -7, -9 supplement

7. **Dairy and Dairy Substitutes:** Yogurt, kiefer, or soy yogurt, 1 cup a day (organic, fat-free)

8. **Fermented Foods:** Sauerkraut, miso, tempeh, sourdough, apple cider vinegar, 1 cup total

9. **Unsalted Seeds:** Flax, hemp, sesame, sunflower seeds, ¼ cup a day

   Unsalted Nuts: Almonds, Brazil nuts, cashews, hazelnuts, pecans, ½ cup a day

10. **"Cell-Friendly" Herbs and Spices:** Garnish entrées and season foods with parsley, rosemary, curry, etc.

 Use Bone-Building Yogurt or Kiefer Daily

Every day try to eat a full cup of plain, unsweetened yogurt or soy yogurt if you have a dairy sensitivity. Yogurt is a fermented product that has been promoted for longevity and has an amazing 452 mg of bioavailable calcium per cup. Yogurt is the most easily digestible and preferred form of dairy. Another source of "friendly bacteria" is kiefer.

Whenever possible, choose organic yogurt, since conventional milk and dairy products often contain residues of growth hormones (used to increase cows' milk production) and antibiotics, which are given to cows to prevent the teat infections (mastitis) caused by the strain of supernormal milk production. Avoid yogurt containing thickeners and stabilizers and use only unsweetened yogurt.

In particular, various "cell-friendly" foods like yogurt and brightly color-coded fruit and vegetables may be a better, economical alternative to maintain better bone health and prevent the onset of osteoporosis than pharmaceutical drugs like bisphophonates.

 Use a Targeted Bone-Building Supplement Daily

Dr. Leticia Rao, Ph.D., emphasizes that there is evidence to show that **we do not absorb more than 500 mg**

of elemental calcium at one time. It is very interesting to note that in nature no food source has more than 500 mg of calcium unless condensed by processing. For example, yogurt contains 452 mg of calcium per cup, whereas non-fat, dry milk powder contains 1,508 mg of calcium per cup. The medical evidence leaves no doubt that the closer your diet and supplements are to the original food source, the closer you and your family are to the bone-building diet designed by your body's ancient architecture.

It's a scientific message of great urgency: The best things you can do for your bones are to eat colorful fruit and vegetables; exercise correctly; and use a bone-building supplement for life insurance. In short, our bones quietly survive and endure our poor diets in a permanent state of lethargy that we accept as "normal" because we can't imagine otherwise. We are unaware that we have the potential to feel better, be smarter, and keep our bones strong—that our bones, when properly nourished, can reach for and achieve more.

Whether you are young, old, or in between, taking a food-based, "targeted" bone-builder supplement can improve your bone, heart, and brain function; improve your mood and memory; and slash the chances of bone or teeth deterioration as you get older.

A Bone-Builder Breakthrough Solution

In 2002, the journal *Food Review* reported on research demonstrating that only four foods—iceberg lettuce, onions, fresh and frozen potatoes, and canned tomatoes—account for 50 percent of our total vegetable consumption. The University of Pennsylvania proved that 60 percent of adult antioxidant intake in 2006 came from coffee.

While obtaining your daily bone-building micronutrient requirements from food would be ideal, the fact
is that many North Americans' diets often fall short of
calcium and many of the other super-critical cofactors.

The Bone-Builder Supplement Solution

Calcium	from citrate-malate, formate, and bisglycinate	500 mg
Magnesium	from aspartate	300 mg
Zinc	from bioactive food base	10 mg
Manganese	from bioactive food base	3 mg
Boron	from the patented OsteoBoron	3 mg
Silicon	from the herb horsetail	3 mg
Copper	from HVP chelate	1 mg
Vitamin D3	natural form cholecalciferol	800 IU
L-lysine	amino acid	400 mg
Vitamin C	from non-acidic calcium ascorbate	100 mg
Lycopene	(a red antioxidant carotenoid from tomatoes)	7 mg
Vitamin B6	(pyridoxine hydrochloride)	10 mg
Vitamin B9	(folate or folic acid)	400 mcg
Selenium	from bioactive food base	100 mcg
Vitamin K1	(menatetrenone) from the "green drink" base	120 mcg
Vitamin B12	(cyanocobalamin)	10 mcg

Note: Elemental calcium means the amount that is absorbed by
your body. The most absorbable forms of calcium are citrate-malate,
formate, and bisglycinate. This formula is highly absorbed in an
alkalinizing "green drink" powdered base that you mix with a
liquid of choice. This formula supports the activity of both types
of bone cells. Both *osteoblast* and *osteoclast* are dramatically enhanced without one being preferentially increased to the detriment
of the other. This formula promotes healthy, balanced bone function
homeostasis and accelerates bone-repair that may have been derailed
because of years of suboptimal bone-building micronutrient intake.

Keep Your Body Moving

In conjunction with excellent food choices and a "molecular-targeted" bone-builder supplement, all of us need to keep our bodies moving.

Before the 1960s, we did not have to worry about getting enough exercise. Our parents and grandparents either walked or rode bicycles to go to work. Parents did not drive their children around. Children and teens biked, walked, and took buses. Children and teens had a daily list of routine chores that had to be done to keep family life harmonious, cooperative, and running smoothly. Today, with hundreds of time-saving conveniences, we have actually become unfit, being too busy and too tired to properly feed and mobilize our faithful, 100 trillion cells!

You need to eat smarter, live smarter, choose smarter, sleep smarter, supplement smarter, and exercise smarter—bringing good nutrition and quality fitness into everything you do.

Fish Oil Supplements Ramp Up Bone-Building

Cholesterol reduction remained the Holy Grail of heart disease medicine until 2004, when elevated, silent inflammation levels, just below the perception of pain, were discovered to be the strongest, problematic component of heart disease, depression, cancer, arthritis, chronic pain, multiple sclerosis, dementia, Alzheimer's, ADD, ADHD, PMS, and osteoporosis. Inflammation is the smoking gun.

The single most important thing you can do to keep silent inflammation under control is this: Daily supplement with ultrapure, high-dose omega-3 fish oils. Fish oils rich in EPA and DHA account for less than

5 percent of all supplement sales and yet they are, along with "green drinks," the most important. Unlike vitamins and minerals, which last only a few hours in the blood-stream, EPA and "bone-smart" DHA long-chain fatty acids from fish oils last several days, so you can take your daily dose all at once if that's easier.

EPA and DHA lower levels of silent inflammation many years before, if not decades before, it advances into any serious health trouble. As an example, Ritalin treats only the symptoms of ADD and ADHD, but omega-3 fish oils treat the underlying cause—silent inflammation. You can test your inflammation status with your physician using the Silent Inflammation Profile (SIP) test, which measures the ratio of arachidonic acid (AA) to EPA in the plasma phospholipids. Nutrasource Diagnostics, associated with the University of Guelph in Ontario, is the testing laboratory and can be reached at (866) 637-8378 in Canada and (800) 404-8171 in the U.S. A good SIP result level is 3.0 and an ideal level is 1.5. Furthermore, reducing sugar consumption lowers excess insulin levels that lower arachidonic acid (AA) formation, lowering your SIP, which ratchets up good bone-building functions.

Important: Be sure to use only pharmaceutical-grade, ultrapure fish oil concentrates tested by the International Fish Oil Standards (IFOS) program administered by the University of Guelph.

Find fish oils that are listed on the IFOS website at www.ifosprogram.com before purchasing any fish oil products, regardless of the advertising claims, since they must meet incredibly rigid IFOS standards for potency, label claim, and purity. Three brands that receive the highest five-star rating on the IFOS website are Genuine Health's entire line of condition-specific, ultrapure omega-3 fish oils, Life Extension's Super EPA-DHA, and Zone Labs Inc.

Do not rely on short-chain essential fatty acids from flaxseed oil, which require nine very difficult biological steps to convert to the long-chain omega-3 essential fatty acids "mood-smart" EPA and "bone-smart" DHA that your body and brain need daily. High-quality fish oils are available in softgels and in liquid form. Leap-frog beyond flaxseed oil and use enteric-coated fish oils that are already long-chain, body-ready, inflammation-lowering, essential fatty acids.

The University of Texas proved that fish oils accelerate healthy bone-building by significantly reducing markers of oxidative stress like urinary F2-isoprostanes.

Fish Oils Found to Aid Bone-Building

A study from the *American Journal of Clinical Nutrition*, dated April 2005, proved the potent power of fish oils rich in EPA and DHA, long-chain omega-3 essential fatty acids. Researchers collected dietary data through a self-administered questionnaire from some 1,500 men and women, aged 45–90. Information on smoking habits, alcohol intake, exercise frequency, reproductive history, and use of vitamins, thyroid hormones, steroids, and estrogen was obtained. Baseline bone mineral density (BMD) was measured. The results show that people with increased consumption of fatty, deep-water fish or fish oil capsules and lower levels of omega-6 fatty acid consumption (corn, sunflower, and sesame oils) had the best BMD results of the hip bones.

Again the *American Journal of Clinical Research*, in November 2004, found that fish or fish oils rich in EPA and DHA increased bone mineral density and strength in the hip bones and spine of both men and women.

Surprisingly, the *Journal of the American College of Nutrition*, in 2005 (Volume 24), found that fish oils reduced inflammation systemically in people with arthritis and increased BMD, which prevented the accelerated development of osteoarthritis.

The Medical University of Southern Africa, Pretoria, South Africa, published very interesting research results in the journal *Prostaglandins and Essential Fatty Acids* (Volume 68, 2003). Their dramatic results explained that fish oils rich in EPA and DHA improved calcium absorption in the small intestine. This is very good news for anyone two years of age or older.

Conclusions

- Fish oils increase calcium absorption, reduce system-wide inflammation, and give a bone-building advantage to your bones. Fish oils rich in "mood-smart" EPA and "bone-smart" DHA are symbiotic with probiotic cultures such as Acidophilus, Lactobacilli, and Bifidobacteria, each helping the other to be absorbed better.

- Dr. Greg M. Cole, Associate Director of the Alzheimer's Disease Research Center at UCLA's School of Medicine, noted that DHA and its metabolic derivative, neuroprotectin D1, reduce the inflammation and toxicity from a gooey, sticky brain toxin called beta amyloid, which is widely believed to contribute to Alzheimer's.

- Studies have found that even low levels of mercury intake from regularly consumed fish can have negative effects on learning and memory in children, teens, and adults. Large fish like grouper, king mackerel, marlin, sea bass, shark, swordfish, and tilefish accumulate significant amounts of mercury, and 90–95 percent is in the highly neurotoxic methylmercury form. The U.S. Food and Drug Administration and Health Canada have issued advisories to limit or avoid these seven fish during pregnancy.

- PCBs (polychlorinated biphenyls) were banned in the 1970s because they increased the risk of cancer. The average level of PCBs in farmed salmon is 36.5 ppb (parts per billion) and 4.7 ppb for wild salmon. It is interesting to note that 95 percent of canned salmon is wild.

- New molecular distillation techniques allow fish oils to be gently purified, removing the heavy metals like mercury, PCBs, and other toxins called dioxins. The take-home message is: Fish oil supplements are safe and the preferred source of crucial EPA and "bone-smart" DHA fatty acids. The preferred sources for fish oils are mackerel, sardines, anchovies, and herring formulated in enteric-coated capsules, for no fishy aftertaste.

Olive Oil for Skin and Bone Health

The right foods act as anti-inflammatory, skin-glowing cosmetics for our facial skin, body skin, and, surprisingly, shiny and lustrous hair and good bones. Food is much more than just a life-sustaining, life-giving, energizing substance. Food is our single most powerful anti-aging tool. The many choices we make daily—or even hourly—immediately influence not only our vital energy and critical mental performance, but also our appearance.

The wrong oils and fats directly influence the growing number of wrinkles and amount of sagging in your face, as well as your drooping skin texture, enlarged pore size, dull skin tone, and undereye bags and puffiness. You can reverse and certainly prevent visible skin damage and put your best face forward by using the oils and salad dressing I use and highly recommend.

Working from the inside out, by using the right oils, the right antioxidants, and quality phytonutrients in natural foods—as well as quality supplements—will also produce striking short-term and cumulative long-term improvements to renew your bones.

I strongly suggest that you incorporate cold-pressed, extra-virgin olive oil into your diet and salad dressing on a daily basis. Olive oil is the type of fat that lowers harmful LDL cholesterol at the same time as it raises the level of heart-protective HDL cholesterol. Olive oil is the only safe, stable oil that does not require refrigeration.

Olive oil contains 75–82 percent of a nonessential monounsaturated fatty acid called oleic acid, a member of the omega-9 family. Oleic acid offers an entire spectrum of beneficial services as it:

- does not readily oxidize, is stable, and does not produce free radicals

- is transported into the cell plasma membrane, helping to maintain the structural integrity of neuronal membranes and bone-building cell membranes

- acts as a regulator in the cell plasma membrane to ensure that EPA- and DHA-rich omega-3 fish oil fats penetrate the cell membrane to keep the lipid bilayer supple, fluid, and stabilized to allow bone-building nutrients to enter bone cells

- helps intestinal absorption of bone-building micro-nutrients
- supports gallbladder activity
- prevents water-retention edema
- reduces the risk of both breast and prostate cancer
- contains antioxidants, in particular the four most powerful polyphenols—tyrosol, hydroxytyrosol, verbascoside, and oleuropein—which are found only in cold-pressed, extra-virgin olive oil and give olive oil its slightly bitter taste; hydroxytyrosol prevents the oxidation (the equivalent of rusting) of keratin protein, the main protein scaffolding in your bones, and protects EPA and "bone smart" DHA fats from peroxidation degradation.

Sam's Savory Salad Dressing

- 2 tbsps per person of cold-pressed, extra-virgin olive oil (organic, if possible)
- 1 tsp of fresh lemon or lime juice to taste or ¾ tsp of unfiltered, unpasteurized apple cider vinegar; alternate between these two
- several drops of both oil of oregano and oil of rosemary
- liberal sprinkle of a salt-free herbal mix seasoning and turmeric
- a dash of flaked or granulated Nova Scotia dulse
- 1 tsp of gomasio (dry-roasted organic sesame seeds)
- 1 clove of finely chopped garlic or a dash of nonirradiated garlic seasoning (garlic is an optional ingredient)
- ½ tsp of clean, pure water
- 1 tbsp of miso

Eat Mindfully

Your mealtimes can be a downtime of comfort, nourishment, and healing or quite the opposite—extremely detrimental. Unfortunately, many people today eat at the same breakneck speed they use for everything else. If you are depressed, anxious, angry, or distracted when eating, your body will not digest or assimilate your food well, and you will not receive the revitalization you need. It is vitally important to switch on a rhythm of mindful calm while eating slowly and savoring your food, and switch off potentially upsetting things like the news, business discussions, or major dilemmas. I am guilty of old eating habits as I tend to eat fast, but I have made an effort to change my eating habits.

I have found that if I say a grace or thanksgiving before my meals or snacks, I slow down my fast-paced rhythm. Grace or a thanksgiving reminds us to be grateful, and to be more conscious of what we eat and how we eat it, using voluntary calorie restriction to keep our energy currency available all life long.

AN ACTION PLAN

Let's condense the information in this book into an action plan for every decade of your life from ages one to 100+ years.

Follow this easy step-by-step guide through each decade of your life. Soon, one decade's dietary strategy will effortlessly be incorporated into the next decade. We are all creatures of habit and we must replace destructive habits with new lifestyle habits, which Dr. Andrew Weil calls a "progressive dietary strategy."

Children One to Five Years

- Start their day with a specially formulated children's supplement, *greens+kids*.

- Encourage active play, especially outside; take them to parks, pools, and the beach.

- Start to focus on unsalted vegetable juices and organic milk rather than pop or sweetened juices. Do not keep candy at home, and avoid processed, fast foods.

- Include unsweetened yogurt and berries in their breakfast protein power shake.

- Have only brightly colored fresh fruit snacks available instead of candy.

- Teach children the difference between "slow food" and "fast food."

- Do not allow children to eat their meals while watching television.

- Daily, work together to make fresh vegetable juice or granola from scratch.

- Do not use regular table salt but introduce them to small amounts of alkalinizing Celtic or Antarctic sea salt; replace peanut butter with unsalted almond butter.

- Remove any Teflon-coated or non-stick pans from your kitchen since they give off a toxic gas, ammonium perfluorooctanoate (C-8), after being heated for two to three minutes. Ninety-five percent of us have C-8 in our blood.

- Have children adopt a few plants. They can be used strategically to improve air quality from "off-gassing" from synthetic materials like carpeting, paint, furniture, and dry cleaning, which give off various toxic emissions that your family breathes in.

The following six plants are easy for children to care for. Encourage them to be plant aware, and bring the outdoors indoors. Good "adoptable" plants are: ferns, palms, carrot tops, pineapple tops, peace lilies, and chrysanthemums.

- Children love to be involved and watch the fermentation of foods. Fermentation makes food more digestible and nutritious. The taste of fermented foods is usually acquired over time. Certain microorganisms can manifest extraordinary culinary transformations into: sauerkraut, kimchi, miso, chutney, yogurt, kiefer, buttermilk, cheese, sour cream, kombucha, sourdough bread, apple cider vinegar, teas, brewed black coffee, microbiotic Japanese pickles or plums, and a Mayan fermented honey called balché. For adults, draft beer and dry red wine are fermented beverages.

- Replace butter with extra-virgin coconut oil (1 tablespoon daily), made by a micro-expelling process.

Children Six to 12 Years

- Start them on one serving daily of an alkalinizing food-based, bone-builder formula mixed in cold cow's, rice, hemp, or almond milk or ½ water and ½ unsweetened juice at breakfast.
- Introduce small amounts of colorful vegetables.
- Make sure they have protein at each meal—start their day with a protein power shake.

- Use yogurt and fresh or frozen berries as desserts.
- Keep "finger foods" like colorful vegetable sticks and a yogurt-based dip handy in the kitchen; do not make candy and pop available.
- Introduce an omega-3 fish oil softgel, or a liquid version, daily for their brains and bones; many pre-adolescents prefer liquid fish oils over softgels.
- Encourage them to join soccer, swimming, baseball, tennis, badminton, gymnastics, snowboarding, volleyball, basketball, or track and field teams.
- Establish a set sleep routine so they get nine full hours of sleep a night.
- Make a salad part of each day and have an automatic, no water, no mold, no hassle sprouter on your kitchen counter so they can grow fresh sunflower, daikon, garlic, and raddish sprouts all year round, even in limited space—just add seeds and water and in four days you can harvest fresh and healthy sprouts. It's that easy!

Teenagers 13–19 Years

- Start their day off with an alkalinizing food-based, bone-building supplement.
- For breakfast, make them a protein power shake—teens love protein smoothies with frozen berries and one or two ice cubes thrown in the blender.
- Encourage them to use three omega-3 fish oil softgels, or 1 tbsp of naturally flavored fish oil liquid every day to elevate moods and increase their motivation, creativity, and learning enthusiasm.

- Include free-range organic eggs from vegetable and flax-fed chickens three times a week, keeping yolks intact.

- Get them involved in planning and preparing ethnic food nights full of colorful salads, vegetables, herbs, and spices; macadamia nut oil is the most stable oil for cooking.

- Keep apple slices, black cherries, raspberries, blueberries, plums, apricots, grapes, and oranges—or slices of melons in season—on the kitchen table for quick snacking.

- Encourage teens to participate in physical education classes each year of high school and join a school sports team.

- For every hour of television, computer, or telephone time, make them equally active in physical activities.

- Limit processed, fast foods, especially sugar and artificial sweeteners.

Those 20–30 Years

- This is a great time to join a gym and go five days a week.

- Use an alkalinizing food-based, bone-building formula daily.

- Start your day with a protein power shake.

- Begin Pilates, Tai Chi, Qigong, spinning, aerobics, taekwon do, martial arts, swimming, or hatha yoga classes once or twice a week—take class action!

- Use three fish oil capsules daily or fish oil liquid for superior bones, brain, and moods.

- If you are pregnant, consult with your health care provider and consider taking a food-based, bone-builder formula twice a day in unsalted vegetable juice if possible.

- Learn about fermentation and eat whole-grain sourdough breads, sauerkraut, yogurt, kiefer, miso, and tempeh. Fermentation boosts digestion and eliminates gas.

- If you drink wine, drink dry red wine in moderation, which contains phytonutrient compounds called salvestrol and resveratrol, doubling the activity of an anti-aging enzyme called sirtuin (Sirt-1). Recent research showed it reduced the flu virus by 98 percent. Salvestrols "trigger" an enzyme protein called CYP1B1 that kills cancer cells.

- If you drink beer, drafts, dark ales, and beers made by the Bavarian (European) beer laws, which do not allow additives. Avoid "light beers," which are full of additives. Always consume alcohol in moderation because it is very hard on your liver and brain cells.

- Read books on physical, emotional, mental, and spiritual health or well-being.

- Do not eat fast foods and drive-thru foods, which support an unhealthy "grab-and-feed" mentality to food.

- If you drink coffee, drink only alkalinizing, un-sweetened coffee and limit coffee to a maximum of 2 cups a day, or try green tea, matcha, white, oolong, or rooibos. The highest-grade green tea is Japanese matcha, which contains up to 137 percent more anti-fat, anti-inflammatory, and anti-cancer amounts of the special polyphenol (phytonutrient) epigallocatechin-3-gallate (EGCG). In 2002, the journal *Phytomedicine* showed that 270 mg of EGCG, plus 3,400 mg of conjugated linoleic acid (CLA), is a potent supplement to speed up abdominal weight loss.

Those 30–40 Years

- Try to exercise five to seven days a week; promote core strength, flexibility, balance, reaction time, and breathing exercises daily; include 30 minutes of weight training daily.
- Use an alkalinizing food-based, bone-building formula daily.
- Use fish oil capsules daily or fish oil liquid for superior bones, brain, and mood.
- Start your day with a protein power shake.
- Walk everywhere you can and ride a bike as much as possible.
- Go hiking and swimming when possible.
- Make time to take an infrared sauna once or twice a week.
- Spend one hour a day in combined prayer and/or meditation.
- This is a great age to stay flexible with hatha yoga, Pilates, Tai Chi, Qigong, martial arts, kayaking, hiking, and stretching.
- Have a big salad every day, use four or five color-coded vegetables at lunch and supper.
- Reduce stress and anxiety with laughter—"laughter is the best medicine."

- Try to go to sleep and rise at the same times at least six days a week.

- Make it a priority to get eight to nine hours of sleep a night.

- Stay close to family and friends, especially your parents and grandparents.

- Try to eat "slow food" not "fast food" (the foods of modern commerce).

- If you eat chocolate, eat only semisweet chocolate that is at least 70 percent cocoa. Eat it at 3:30 p.m. to raise the "feel good" hormones serotonin and beta-endorphins.

Those 40–60 Years

- Be enthusiastic about your daily exercise, especially the bone-building core exercises in Chapter 9. Do include weight-resistance training three times a week.

- Get outside daily, doing chores, a work project, or exercise in the sunlight.

- Use an alkalinizing food-based, bone-building supplement daily before breakfast and again before supper, which will ensure that you receive 1,000 mg of elemental calcium.

- Start your day with a protein power shake.

- Use fish oil capsules daily or fish oil liquid for superior bones, brain, and mood.

- Consider a massage and infrared sauna once a week.

- Say a grace or thanksgiving before all meals and snacks.

- Eat three balanced meals a day and a 10:30 a.m. snack and a 4:30 p.m. snack.
- Drink eight glasses of water a day.
- Drink green tea daily.

Those 60+ Years

- Daily have one or two predigested whey isolate protein power shakes with berries.
- Use an alkalinizing food-based, bone-builder formula twice a day.
- Use three capsules of omega-3 fish oils or a liquid version daily for superior bones.
- Stay involved with an exercise class at least five times a week to stay lean and strong.
- Consider watching only a maximum of one or two hours of television per day.
- Spend one to two hours a day in quiet reflection, prayer, or meditation.
- Laugh lots and read more.
- Walk everywhere you can; be outdoors; use stairs, not an elevator.
- Consider DHEA and melatonin restorative, natural, bioidentical hormone replacement therapy with transdermal creams or sublingually.
- Chew your foods well and do not eat while watching television.
- Try an omega-3, -6, -7, and -9 essential oil supplement daily as an insurance policy.
- Volunteer some time to a cause in your community— be a wise elder!

You can use Bone-Builder Tip 1 and make the one-minute protein power shake for breakfast and again at supper. It is predigested, liquid, and outrageously delicious.

My Italian father, affectionately called Papa Joe, in his nineties, would make an alkalinizing high-alpha whey protein power shake with frozen berries once or twice a day. The frozen berries make the protein power shake refreshingly cool, tasty, and nutritious.

There is an old Italian expression he used to love to repeat to me: "*Chi vuol viver sano e lesto beve scotta e cena presto,*" which translates as, "If you want to live a healthy and happy life, drink whey and dine early." I can still hear the beautiful echo of Papa Joe's voice literally singing these words. Salute, Papa Joe, you were a wise elder!

BE BONE WISE DURING EVERY DECADE OF YOUR LIFE

We cheat our infants, children, and teens of bone-building foods and supplements. Of course, not all the scientific information is in, but more than enough is known to point to the right color-coded foods and "molecular-targeted" supplements that can make a dramatic difference in preserving the magnificence of our most precious structural asset—our skeletal system.

Antioxidant authority Dr. Lester Packer, at the University of California, Berkeley, recommends that it's much smarter to consume a broad range of color-coded antioxidant polyphenols instead of just focusing on one, he says, because they do not work in isolation: Their bone-building protecting powers are much stronger when they work together. For example, thrilling new research at Tufts University gives a glimpse of the power of the polyphenol antioxidants in color-coded foods to rev up bone-building functions and even reverse bone-breakdown. It's mind-boggling to think that brightly colored, "cell-friendly" fruit and vegetables can rejuvenate you and your family's bones all life long—yet true!

The Lure of the 100-Mile Diet

There is a fast growing group of people called "locavores," self-styled concerned culinary adventurers, who for the months of May, June, July, August, September, and October, one-half of the year, pledge not to eat any fresh berries, fruit, salad, or vegetables unless they are grown within 100 miles (160 kilometers) of their home. Doing this supports local farmers instead of the vast monoculture, corporate agribusiness. Consumers seeking to eat ethically and preserve farmland around their cities are embracing locally grown, seasonal food as the eco-healthy choice.

The most important thing to remember is that your nails, teeth, heart, arteries, brain, and bones are growing and changing every second. Bones are living tissue that thrive on the right diet; smart bone-building supplementation; exercise; stimulation from sunshine, producing vitamin D3; and the essential vitamin K1 from green vegetables.

It is never too early or too late to shape or reshape your own or your family's bone destiny—to actually encourage growth of new strong bone cells for a lifetime!

Healthy bones, healthy life, healthy you!

Part II

A Physician's Perspective on Bone-Building

Written by: Dr. Carolyn DeMarco, M.D.,
Practicing Physician and Woman Specialist

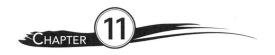

CHAPTER 11

Put Your Bones to the Test

This book offers insight and hope that will allow you to actually prevent needless fractures, "dowager's hump," and loss of mobility or independence, and even regain enough bone mass to take you out of the high-risk zone. Both bone health development and maintenance are natural and spontaneous when you follow this book's simple but comprehensive program. I personally follow it!

And perhaps most importantly, the life-saving information and guidelines provided in *The Bone-Building Solution* will keep your bones strong and maintain your bone mass, so that you can avoid the need for prescription drugs altogether.

Naturally, people in their later years or those who have already experienced a fracture due to osteoporosis, may need a medication to assist them, but the majority of us can naturally prevent and to some extent even reverse osteoporosis.

I present chapters 11 and 12 to you so you can fully understand the typical medical approach that most physicians utilize. These chapters will also show you how to make educated choices about both testing and treatment, and how to combine the best of natural approaches with the best of medication based solutions.

No matter what positive changes or fine-tuning you decide to make in your diet, exercise, supplement, and lifestyle practices, give yourself at least eight full weeks to truly adapt and assimilate the changes. Remember, you are undoing years of eating habits and a lifestyle that may not have been good for your health. You are also acquiring new tastes, new foods, and a better way of living. I have never met anyone who regretted making the health optimizing and rejuvenating changes that you will find clearly outlined throughout this book.

I know, as a physician, that osteoporosis is preventable. I also know that it has reversal potential. This book is an invitation to take care of your own optimum well-being and to give you real hope that you can have healthier bones, a stronger stature, better posture, and more fluid biomechanical movement naturally, all life long.

PUT YOUR BONES TO THE TEST

Osteopenia

Many people are distressed to learn they have osteopenia, but it should just be considered as a warning sign, a kind of biological "wake-up call."

Osteopenia implies that your bone mass is low, but still within the normal range. The current trend is to replace the term osteopenia with the clearer and more precise terms, "low bone mass" or "low bone density." Osteopenia is not a disease. In fact, all men and women would be diagnosed with osteopenia if they lived long enough.

Osteopenia means that your bone density could fall anywhere between the lower fifth to sixteenth percentile compared to the average young normal bone mineral density (BMD). Even in people who are 25 or 30, this is still normal. Furthermore, the osteopenia diagnosis does not take into account body size or other major risk factors.

Smaller people will appear to have lower BMD automatically because the way bones are measured doesn't correct for their small bone dimension. Therefore, some measurements that fall in the osteopenic range may be there in part due to small body size and small bone size.

Osteoporosis Is Not an Isolated Disease

Osteoporosis is not a dreadful disease that randomly strikes some of us. Weak bone structure does not happen suddenly and without cause; and the causes of osteoporosis are often associated with a poor diet, a lack of proper exercise, low total calcium and vitamin D intake, daily consumption of pop and acidifying junk food, excessive stress, smoking, medication use (especially steroids), a strong family history of osteoporosis, previous low impact fracture, alcohol abuse, and toxic exposure. I collectively call these the *bone depleting factors*. Our unhealthy lifestyle habits deplete our bones of their precious stores of life-supportive minerals. The ultimate price we pay for excesses in these destructive modern-day, "grab-and-feed" habits is porous, weak bones that deteriorate into osteoporosis.

In reviewing the available anthropological data from around the world, I discovered that osteoporosis occurs in some countries more than it does in others, although this is rapidly changing as developing countries adapt Western eating habits and sedentary lifestyles. Canada and the United States have some of the highest osteoporosis rates in the world. In 1992, *The Proceedings of the Society of Experimental Biology & Medicine* printed research that showed the incidence of hip fractures in the Japanese, even in the elderly, is almost 60 percent less than in North America.

Our fast-paced, stressful lifestyle leaves us too exhausted to exercise or even prepare healthy food. Our lack of healthy food and eating patterns, exercise, stress reduction, deep natural sleep, and bone-building supplementation cause a lifelong pattern of bone destruction for ourselves and for our children.

Prevent a Future Shock

I'm not suggesting that it is easy to change the patterns of a lifetime, or that you can simply stop taking necessary medications because they increase your risk of developing osteoporosis. However, it is important to be aware of some of the most important risk factors you can change with simple, effective, and safe lifestyle adjustments, proper exercise, and a smart supplement action plan, regardless of your age. For more detailed information on each of these risk factors, please visit my website at www.demarcomd.com

12 Risk Factors You Can Change

1. Not having your BMD tested if indicated, i.e., if you are a man or woman under 65 who has serious risk factors; or, because risk increases dramatically with age, if you are a woman over 65 or a man over 70

2. Lack of weight bearing exercises, weight training (including exercises targeted to strengthen the back, hip and wrist or other problem areas), as well as balance and core strengthening exercises

3. Smoking

4. Over consumption of alcohol

5. Over consumption of caffeine

6. Low calcium and vitamin D3 intake or supplementation

7. Low body weight

8. Taking certain medications

9. High table salt intake

10. High sugar intake, including pop and colas

11. Not fall-proofing your house

12. Overall poor nutrition, especially an acidifying diet that leads to consistent bone deterioration

The good news is that by following the well-documented recommendations and step-by-step self-help action plan, outlined in chapters 1 to 10 of this groundbreaking book, you can experience lifelong bone health naturally. It is only through major changes to our lifestyle—including diet, exercise, and stress reduction that we can truly hope to prevent and reverse osteoporosis. Even if you already have osteoporosis and have experienced a low impact or fragility fracture, lifestyle changes are the major preventative tactic and are at least as important, if not more important, than medication in any treatment management protocol.

When Should You Have a Bone Density Test?

- All postmenopausal women under 65 who have one major risk factor should be tested. These risk factors include low-impact fracture (also known as fragility fractures), low-trauma spinal compression fracture, family history of osteoporosis (especially maternal hip fracture), taking steroids continuously for three or more months, premature menopause (before age 45), malabsorption syndrome, or over-activity of the parathyroid gland. Low-trauma fractures are caused by forces that would usually not break a bone, such as a fall from the standing position. Postmenopausal women under 65 should also be tested if they have two minor risk factors, including taking medications such as Coumadin, anticonvulsants or heparin, low dietary intake of calcium, smoking, excessive caffeine intake (more than 4 cups a day), a weight of less than 57 kg (or 10 percent less than at age 25), or a history of rheumatoid arthritis.

- Any situation where the bone density measurement would make a difference in whether or not a treatment was started.

- All women 65 or older regardless of risk factors.

- All men 70 or older (under 60 if you have any of the major risk factors previously mentioned).

- All men, women, and children who have known secondary causes of osteoporosis, which means osteoporosis due to other medical conditions, or medications used to treat these illnesses.

Bone Density Testing—Info You Need to Know

Bone mineral density (BMD) tests measure the amount of minerals in a specific area of bone. The more minerals, the denser the bone appears on the X-ray scan. Bone mineral density testing is the most practical and cost effective testing method currently available, but it only measures bone at two sites, the hip and the spine, and tells us nothing about bone strength and architecture.

As New Zealand health activist Gillian Sanson says in her book, *The Myth of Osteoporosis*, "the fact is that you may have low bone density and never fracture. Or you may have normal or better than normal bone density and still have a fracture."

A new technique known as high definition peripheral QCT can give detailed information about the structure and strength of both cortical and trabecular bone. However, the major drawback to this test is that it exposes the patient to 50 times more radiation than the commonly used DEXA test. It measures the bone density in the forearm and wrist and currently is only used in research.

Bone density can vary throughout the 206 bones in your skeleton. There is increased recognition that non-vertebral, non-hip fractures are also important and can cause as much disability as hip fractures. Other sites include the wrist, the ribs, the pelvis, clavicle, and humerus.

The preferred medical procedure for osteoporosis testing is via a dual-energy X-ray absorptiometry test (DEXA). However, ultrasound densitometry is a quick and inexpensive screening technique that can be available in doctors' offices, pharmacies, or shopping malls.

The site most commonly measured is the heel. The results strongly correlate with fracture risk but are no substitute for DEXA. It will let you know if you are in a high-risk category and need to get a DEXA scan. For more detailed information on BMD scans, and other testing modalities please refer to my website at www. drdemarco.com. One important piece of advice is to make sure you have your bone scans done at the same time of year and on the same machine, if possible.

There is currently an effort to try and standardize the reading and reporting of bone density. The International Society for Clinical Densitometry has issued official guidelines to help eliminate inaccuracies due to a lack of proper standardization of machines used. These can be viewed at www.ISCD.org. There is currently no agreed-upon international reference standard and each manufacturer establishes its own data, resulting in *completely different standards* between various DEXA machines measuring the same bone!

Accuracy of diagnosis is fundamental and crucial for diagnosing osteoporosis and re-evaluating the effectiveness and safety of a treatment protocol over the years. The National Women's Health Network publication, *Osteoporosis Fact Sheet*, suggests that a better evaluation of bone density is obtained by comparing a person's bone to that of other fracture-free, healthy people of the same age, as opposed to the current practice of comparing to a young person's bone at the peak of its density.

There are further concerns with regard to BMD testing. According to many experts, the following are some of the most important limits of bone density that the public should be made aware of:

1. BMD measurement is not an ideal measure of true bone strength. Bone quality is not only determined by bone mass, but also by the micro-architecture of the bone. The porosity, brittleness, the crystal size and shape, the scaffolding structure of the collagen proteins, the ability to rapidly repair micro-fractures, the connectivity and shape of the trabecular (interior honeycomb) bone, and the vasculature network of blood vessels' ability to carry sufficient supplies of bone-building micronutrients all influence the quality and the quantity of our 206 bones. There is currently no test available to the public that can measure bone strength and give you accurate information about the micro-architecture of your bones.

2. It should be used after correction for body size and/or bone size, age, sex, and local variations in average bone mineral density.

3. It should not be considered the sole indicator of present and future fracture risk, but only one risk factor that should be measured in terms of the whole picture of your lifestyle and environmental risks.

The Advisory Committee for Guidelines and Protocols for Bone Density Measurement in Women in the province of British Columbia, Canada put it this way: "Low bone density is only one of the many factors that can increase the risk of fracture."

The committee goes on to say that indiscriminate bone density testing and needless treatment of osteopenia may be examples of the medical intervention of natural processes such as menopause and aging. "Medicalization" means treating natural processes like diseases, and relying heavily on highly technological medical treatment when less invasive approaches could be just as beneficial. However, bone density testing can still provide valuable information and help people decide when hormone or drug treatment may be beneficial.

What is important to understand is that while bone density testing has limitations, it remains a useful, non-invasive procedure that can indicate whether or not osteoporosis is affecting any of your 206 bones.

Many physicians continue to emphasize solely the single risk factor—low bone density. However, it is now clear that the causes of bone fractures are complex, and blaming them on low density is not scientifically valid.

In an effort to target treatment to those who need it the most, and to avoid over-treating those at low risk, most osteoporosis groups now recommend looking at the BMD measurement only in the larger context of the person's overall health, nutritional status, and major risk factors.There is no substitute for taking early preventive measures if you are even at the slightest risk of developing osteoporosis. Talk to your doctor, and if you decide that BMD testing is appropriate, consider the test results as only one marker for the possibility of osteoporosis.

Male Osteoporosis: Under-Diagnosed and Poorly Studied

On behalf of the International Osteoporosis Foundation, at www.osteofound.org, Dr. Ego Seeman, Melbourne Professor of Medicine and osteoporosis expert, has written an excellent paper on the subject, including an osteoporosis risk test for men.

"Most men, most doctors and most governments are not aware of the problem of osteoporosis in men," says Seeman. "When a male patient enters the doctor's office, the doctor thinks of heart disease, cholesterol problems, blood pressure and strokes, sometimes prostate, lung or bowel cancer, but osteoporosis and fractures—never or rarely….[Yet] the lifetime risks of a man suffering an osteoporotic fracture is greater than his likelihood of developing prostate cancer."

Men pay a higher price for their fractures. Although fragility fractures are less common in men than in women, when they occur these fractures are associated with a disability and death rate higher than in women.

HOW TO INTERPRET YOUR TEST RESULTS

The results of a bone density test can be confusing at first, but once you know how to interpret the numbers and graphs, you'll find the results very informative. Each bone normally has a different bone density. In order to standardize results across different sites and technologies, bone density measures are usually reported as T-Scores and Z-Scores. These scores have caused much confusion and misinterpretation among doctors, as well as patients.

What Is a T-Score?

T-Scores are calculated from an individual's bone density results, the variation in bone density measurement, and the average bone density of a young normal reference population at peak bone mass. The age of the young normal reference population used to determine

references for T-Scores differs among different manufacturers of bone density measurement devices, but is
usually between 20 and 35 years of age. This is the age
range when bone density is at its peak and osteoporosis-
related fracture risk is at its lowest. Results are expressed
as standard deviation (SD) scores above or below the
average measurement for the young normal. A T-Score
of –2 indicates that the person's score is 2 standard
deviations below average for a young normal person
of the same gender. On average, every T-Score above
or below 0 represents about 10–15 percent reduction (or
increase) in bone mass. For example a T score of -2 in
the spine means that the person's bone mass is about 20
per cent lower in the spine than the average for a young
normal person of the same gender.

Osteoporosis is defined by the T-Score, as originally
decided by the World Health Organization (WHO) in
1992. A T-Score of –2.5 or lower indicates the presence of
osteoporosis. An intermediate condition, called osteopenia or low bone mass, is defined as a T-Score between –1
and –2.5. The WHO criteria were designed as descriptive
terms in order to determine the prevalence of bone mass
at different levels in different populations. These cut-off
points were never intended to be used as treatment cut-
off points (i.e., to decide whether to treat or not). It turns
out that the osteoporosis cut-off point actually makes
some biological sense; the risk of fracture is substantially
increased at –2.5, and the majority of people do not reach
this level until they are in their eighties. Furthermore,
–2.5 seems to be the T-Score at which treatment, at least
with bisphosphonates, the most commonly prescribed
drugs, consistently work.

In contrast to *osteoporosis*, though, *osteopenia* is not as useful a term in determining who should be treated and who should not. In fact some experts maintain that comparing bone density, which normally and naturally decreases with age without necessarily leading to an increase in fracture rate, is creating a falsely elevated rate of osteopenia, thus causing much unnecessary anxiety.

"Using the WHO standards," says the British Columbia Office of Health Technology Assessment, "22 percent of all women over age 50 will be defined as having osteoporosis and 52 percent as having osteopenia. Therefore the resulting epidemic observed in the last few years is more apparent than real." Therefore, it is also useful to compare your bone density to that of your own age group, and ethnic group, which is what the Z-Score is all about.

What Is a Z-Score?

We usually lose bone as we age, so our T-Scores normally drop. The Z-Score presents our BMD in a different way, as a comparison with people our own age. A low Z-Score is a warning that we're losing bone more rapidly than our peers, so we need to be monitored more closely by our doctor. The Z-Score compares a person's results to those of an average reference population of the same age and gender (as opposed to the T-Score, which compares the patient's measurement to that of a young population at peak bone mass). Just as for the T-Score, the Z-Score also takes into account the variability in the normal age-matched population. The results are expressed as positive or negative scores, referring to measurements above or below the average for the reference population.

A score between –2 and +2 includes 95 percent of the population. Therefore, if you have a –2, you are in the lower fifth percentile for your age. If you have a Z-Score of +2, you are in the highest ninety-fifth percentile for your age. A score of 0 means that the person's bone density is exactly average for age and gender.

For every reduction in the Z-Score, the risk of fracture increases approximately twofold. That is, if the person's Z-Score is –1, his or her risk of fracture is twice that of the average person at his or her age; for a score of –2, the person's risk of fracture is four times higher than the average person's; for a score of –3, the person's risk of fracture is six times higher than the average. These differences are called relative risk; we ascertain one person's risk compared to the average person's.

BETTER WAYS FOR DOCTORS TO MEASURE UP TO OSTEOPOROSIS

Groundbreaking Research

Dr. Steven Cummings, at the University of California, San Francisco, in *The New England Journal of Medicine* in 1995, explained that low bone density *combined with* a high number of known osteoporosis risk factors is the very best predictor of osteoporotic fracture. They found nearly 24 factors important for predicting the risk of hip fracture.

In this very sophisticated study, Dr. Cummings discovered that bone density and 17 other risk factors are especially meaningful indicators of osteoporosis hip fracture risk and increase the chance of breaking a hip by 50–100 percent.

The 17 Independent Risk Factors for Hip Fracture Your Doctor Must Consider

According to Dr. Steven Cummings, the people with the lowest bone density in their age group and the greatest number of the 17 risk factors are at greatest risk. *Doctors are to interpret bone density measurements, hand in hand, equally with each patient's personal risk factors.* The 17 risk factors are:

1. Advancing age
2. Low bone density
3. Being taller at age 25 than today
4. Current caffeine intake
5. Previous hyperthyroidism
6. Any fracture since age 50
7. Poor overall self-rated health
8. Poor distance depth perception
9. Weighing less than you did at age 25
10. Current use of anticonvulsant drugs
11. Lack of exercise, as in not walking daily for exercise
12. Low-frequency hearing loss and impaired vision
13. A resting pulse of 80 beats or more per minute
14. Tendency to stand on feet less than four hours a day
15. The inability to rise from a chair without using your arms
16. A history of maternal hip fracture (especially if your mother fractured a hip before age 80)
17. Current use of long-acting benzodiazepines (tranquilizers, sleeping medications, and anti-anxiety drugs)

In a paper presented at the May 2006 World Congress on Osteoporosis, the World Health Organization Collaborating Center in the UK tackled the question of whom would benefit most from treatment and how to best optimize fracture risk prediction. They consulted the results of 12 studies comprising 250,000 person-years of observation and 3,500 fractures.

Additionally, there is a simplified list of *seven* factors that contribute to increased fracture risk independent of BMD. These include age, previous fragility fracture, a family history of fracture, rheumatoid arthritis, lack of exercise, alcohol use, and the use of oral steroids. By targeting these seven risk factors, doctors can quickly access fracture risk in an individual and, combined with the results of the BMD testing, determine those who would most benefit from treatment.

Furthermore, the practical utility of examining these simple seven risk factors has been validated in research on 230,000 people followed for 1.2 million person-years.

The New Urine and Blood Tests for Bone-Building and Bone-Breakdown

Currently, there are several urine tests that detect excess bone-breakdown and help to address the future risk of osteoporosis. Also, these non-invasive urine tests can help determine the success of your prevention or treatment program.

The Type 1 collagen test examines the excretion of protein fragments from bone in the urine. Bone-breakdown requires a breakdown of this protein. The more protein fragments in the urine, the more rapid the systemic bone-breakdown and the clearer the indication that bone quality is suboptimal. Bone changes slowly over years, but bone turnover can change in as little as six weeks.

1. The first test is called the n-telopeptide (NTX) or the c-telopeptides (CTX) Osteomark Test for Telopeptides of Type 1 Collagen, which measures the levels of bone-breakdown in urine. NTX levels can also be measured in the blood.

2. The second test involves the measurement of the collagen cross-links, pyridinium and deoxypyridinium (PYD or DPD). As bones break down, they are released in the urine. Higher than normal levels of pyridinium and deoxypyridinium cross-links in the urine indicate an increased rate of bone-breakdown.

3. We also look at the deoxypyridinium to creatinine ratio because it is very specific to bone-breakdown. The pyridinium to creatinine ratio reflects both cartilage breakdown as well as bone-breakdown. Creatinine is a blood or urine test that reflects kidney function.

4. There are also blood tests that measure the rate of bone formation. This is associated with high levels of bone-building proteins in bone such as osteocalcin. Bone-specific alkaline phosphatase (ALP) helps form new calcium crystals in bones, and blood levels of this bone enzyme give an indication of new bone formation.

These accurate and inexpensive urine tests reveal rapid bone loss. But, just like bone density measurements, what "normal values" the laboratories choose to use is important. Recent studies have helped to determine that the "normal values" being used are reasonable. These tests do not take the place of bone density testing, but they do add information that bone density testing cannot provide.

Bone-turnover marker levels can also be used to determine whether bone-building supplements and / or medical treatments are working. It is ideal to have each sample obtained at approximately the same time of day, preferably in the early morning, since the average levels fluctuate over the course of a day or night. These markers can help determine the dynamic, living status of your 206 bones, and help confirm that your treatment is working.

What Your Doctor May Not Know

The level of awareness about osteoporosis diagnosis and treatment is growing every day. However, there could still be substantial improvement in diagnosis, treatment, and in careful follow-up of all those who have had a low impact fracture.

Some doctors still make recommendations and medication decisions on the sole basis of the outcome of the DXA or DEXA bone density scan, and some prescribe medication based on the questionable diagnosis of osteopenia alone.

My research reaffirms my position that by making wise lifestyle, exercise, diet, and bone-building supplement choices, you can successfully prevent, treat, and reverse most cases of weak bones and osteoporosis naturally.

The miracle of the human body is that many, if not all, of these conditions can be turned around—literally reversed. Your superior bone health and biomechanical movement can be restored.

We can cool the fires of accelerated bone loss simply by eliminating its causes and adding "cell-friendly" foods, as well as a bone-building supplement to our menu makeover. In this book, we have tried to provide a clear formula for the significant reduction of osteoporosis, loss of stature, poor posture, and a loss of fluid biomechanical movement—and the recovery of your overall good health. Adopt the comprehensive step-by-step action plan in this book and change your life!

INVEST IN YOUR BONES—STAND TALL

What began as a "thinking about" osteoporosis project on my part turned into an in-depth, comprehensive" rethinking" of the nature and causes of excessive bone-breakdown and loss of fluid biomechanical movement. My rethinking is now calling for a new, fresh, "open window" approach that will enable you to keep your bone structure and function healthy and strong for a lifetime.

Just as a stray sentence could cause confusion in this paragraph, a stray trans fat, excess sugar, or processed food molecule can create havoc if it lands in the wrong place, and there is no way to control where it ends up. These stray molecules accumulate, and eventually they can cause your bones to disintegrate.

Today, proper exercise, a smart diet, and a biocompatible bone-building supplement promise to yield the greatest bone health benefits within months.

CHAPTER 12

The Pros and Cons of Medication

MEETING YOUR BONES' NUTRITIONAL NEEDS IS A TOP PRIORITY

You are now aware that your bones and joints are alive and maintain a complex and dynamic process of growth that requires daily, high-quality nutrition. It is startling that the daily nutritional needs of our bones are almost totally ignored, even by those highest at risk for osteoporosis. It is even more puzzling that men and women are regularly advised to supplement with calcium alone or, at best, calcium with vitamin D3, which is not sufficient for a bone-building supplement. Furthermore, some physicians do not understand the benefits of reducing acidifying foods in patients' diets or ramping up metabolic exercise to stimulate healthy new bone tissue growth at any or every age.

Dr. Randall Stafford, M.D., Ph.D., of Stanford University Prevention Research Center, commented, "Physicians and patients may be so enamoured with the new drugs available today that they are neglecting calcium, this very important component of osteoporosis treatment."

Dr. Stafford continues, "Greater attention to osteoporosis is critical and this includes vitamin D3, calcium and cofactors, and physical activity."

Bone Medications: Fraught with Uncertainties

If you are diagnosed with osteoporosis, your physician will likely recommend medication to reduce your risk of fracture. If you are diagnosed with the more imprecise condition of osteopenia, which is a gray zone with less clear-cut answers, your doctor should certainly recommend a bone-building supplement and an exercise program to reduce your risk of developing osteoporosis. If you have osteopenia, the decision on whether to start medication will depend on your age and current bone density, how your bone density has changed over time (if the information is available), and your risk factor profile. If these elements indicate that your risk of developing osteoporosis is high, then taking a drug plus lifestyle intervention may be the best option. If, on the other hand, you have no or very few risk factors, you could consider lifestyle changes including diet, exercise, and a food-based, bone-building supplement *without* prescription medication.

I discuss the drugs that are currently approved for the prevention or treatment of osteoporosis, for whom and for what conditions they are approved, how well they work, and their side effects in great detail on my website at www.drdemarco.com. You should be aware, however, that although many of these drugs can effectively reduce fracture rates by up to 50 percent, *none* are 100 percent effective. Thus, you need to consider all of the factors that contribute to fracture risk and ensure that you follow a comprehensive program that includes core-balancing exercise and a food-based, bone-building supplement. The information contained in this chapter and throughout the book will help you and your physician create such a program.

MEDICATED TREATMENTS FOR OSTEOPOROSIS

All of the currently approved drugs reduce fracture rates by increasing bone density and reducing rates of bone turnover. Osteoporosis results from either increased bone loss or decreased bone formation. All but two of the currently approved drugs work by reducing the amount of bone lost such that a net gain in bone density occurs over time. The drugs that reduce bone loss render ineffective the bone cells that break down bone. The two drugs that form new bone are thought to stimulate bone-forming cells, as well as to inhibit resorption of bone, but the precise action of these drugs is still unknown. The currently approved classes of drugs are categorized as bisphosphonates, estrogen replacement or hormone replacement therapies, selective estrogen receptor modulators (SERMs), and anabolic agents (parathyroid hormone and strontium ranelate).

Currently, because of their ability to reduce fracture risk at both the hip and spine, bisphosphonates are the most widely prescribed drugs for treating osteoporosis. Bisphosphonates work by being absorbed onto bone crystals. When these bone crystals are taken up by the cells that break down bone (the osteoclasts), they stop the osteoclasts from working, and thus prevent further breakdown or resorption.

There are two main drugs in this category—Fosamax (or alendronate), which has been studied for ten years; and Actonel (or risedronate), which has been studied for five to seven years. In the United States a new bisphosphonate known as bonviva (or ibandronate) can be given either daily or once a month.

All bisphosphonates may irritate the esophagus and cause irritation and indigestion if not taken according to exact instructions. Severe bone and joint pain is a rare side effect as is osteonecrosis or death of the jawbone.

Health advocate Gillian Sanson, in her book, *The Myth of Osteoporosis*, warns that bisphosphonates stay in bone for more than ten years, and halting treatment does not remove them from the body. Furthermore, these drugs disrupt the mechanism that allows the osteoclasts to remove old weakened bone so that the osteoblast cells can build new bone. With the shutting down of the osteoclasts by bisphosphonates, the osteoblasts (bone-builders) may become immobilized.

Some evidence suggests that this suppression of bone remodeling may reduce bone toughness and increase bone fragility. Dr. Seeman also cautions, "Over time this process may produce a thinned and brittle structure prone to failure."

Experts disagree on how long to continue the bisphosphonates. Some, like Seeman, advocate cutting the dose in half after 10 years, while others, like Dr. Susan Ott, limit the length of treatment to five years.

You must do your own research into drug options and discuss your questions and concerns with your doctor.

Classes of Drugs	Approved for	The Pros	The Cons
Bisphosphonates (Actonel, Fosamax, Bonviva)	Postmenopausal osteoporosis; postmenopausal bone loss; male bone loss; glucosteroid-induced osteoporosis in men and women	Large increase in bone density at hip and spine; reduces spine and hip fractures by up to 50 percent	Small risk of upper GI side effects and severe joint and muscle pain, and osteonecrosis (death of the jawbone) especially with intravenous forms
ERT/HRT	Postmenopausal bone loss	Modest increase in bone density; reduces spine and hip fractures by up to 30 percent Relieves menopausal symptoms	Increased risk of stroke and heart attack, blood clotting, gallbladder attacks, slight increase in breast cancer risk
SERMs (Evista)	Postmenopausal bone loss	Modest increase in spine bone density, preserves hipbone density; reduces spine fractures by up to 50 percent; reduction in breast cancer and "bad" LDL cholesterol	No effect on hip fractures; increase in hot flashes, blood clotting risk, studied for only three years

(Continue on page 326)

(Continued from page 325)

Classes of Drugs	Approved for	The Pros	The Cons
Synthetic hormone: Calcitonin (*Miacalcin, Calcimar*)	Postmenopausal osteoporosis; painful spinal fractures; also useful for men	Modest increase in spine bone density and reduction in spine fractures by up to 36 percent; pain relief for spine fractures	No effect on hipbone density or fractures
Synthetic hormone: Parathyroid hormone (*Forteo*) and Preos	Men and women with severe osteoporosis and high risk of fracture	Potential large increase in spine bone density by 8–10 percent	Little to no effect on hipbone density; ability to reduce hip or spine fractures not tested; can be used for only two years; has to be given by daily self injection; very expensive; concern re: causing rare bone cancer in mice
Strontium Ranelate	Post-menopausal osteoporosis; post-menopausal bone loss; and male bone loss	Increases bone density at the hip and spine; decreases vertebral and non vertebral fractures	Few side effects; possible low risk of increased blood clotting

PROMISING NEW TREATMENTS

RANK Ligand Inhibitors

Cutting edge research is being done into agents that can inhibit a substance known as RANK Ligand. This substance enhances the activity of osteoclasts. Among the modalities being studied is a vaccine to Rank Ligand and denosumab (formerly known as AMG 162) a human antibody to RANK Ligand. According to Dr. Marjorie Luckey at the Mount Sinai School of Medicine in New York, phase one and two studies on denosumab show that it causes rapid sustained and reversible decreases in bone turnover. So far no serious side effects have been demonstrated. Other modalities based on new understandings of the bone cell biology are also being developed.

Strontium Ranelate

Strontium is an abundant natural element found in the earth's crust and seawater. According to Dr. Alan Gaby in his book, *Preventing and Reversing Osteoporosis*, the human body contains 320 mg of strontium, nearly all of which is in bone and connective tissues. Gaby cites studies that indicate that strontium may have a significant role in the prevention and treatment of osteoporosis and other bone diseases, particularly metastatic bone cancer.

Strontium ranelate (trade name is Protelos) reduces the incidence of vertebral fractures in postmenopausal women with low bone density. The precise mechanism of bone changes resulting from strontium ranelate treatment have not yet been elucidated, but, like parathyroid hormone (PTH), strontium ranelate appears to decrease bone resorption and stimulate bone formation at the same time.

Researchers conducted a recent three-year trial of 1,649 women, most of whom had a previous fracture. After three years, 139 had a new vertebral fracture in the treatment group compared with 222 in the placebo group. There did not appear to be any significant adverse effects.

In a new trial whose results were presented in August 2005, strontium ranelate was found to reduce the incidence of non-vertebral fractures including hip fractures over a three-year period. This form of strontium has now been approved for the treatment of osteoporosis in many European countries and in Australia. Strontium also was shown to have demonstrated an early and sustained reduction over five years in both vertebral and non-vertebral fractures in women over the age of 80. Protelos reduces the risk of vertebral fracture by 31 percent and non-vertebral fractures by 26 percent.

It is unclear whether other forms of strontium, such as strontium citrate, have the same effect on bone, because no research has been done on the other forms of strontium.

It is important not to take calcium and strontium at the same time because strontium inhibits calcium absorption.

PROMISING NATURAL TREATMENTS

Human Growth Hormone

Human growth hormone (hGH) is the most abundant hormone made by the pituitary gland in the brain. It hits

its peak during the rapid growth phase of adolescence, and then steadily declines as we age. Until recently hGH was difficult to obtain and very expensive. However, in the mid-1980s two drug companies were able to produce hGH through recombinant DNA technology, making it widely available for research and treatment. Human growth hormone may have an important role in the treatment of osteoporosis. It increases bone remodeling and may be useful during late post-menopause or post-andropause. It is another treatment that could be useful for both men and women. Much more research is still needed.

The Role of Progesterone in Bone Health

Thanks to the pioneering work of University of British Columbia professor, Dr. Jerilynn Prior, the critical role of progesterone in bone health has been brought to the forefront.

There has been some evidence that progesterone enhances the formation of new bone. Progestins (progestagens), used in HRT and contraceptives, have been reported to prevent or reverse bone loss in certain clinical situations. Dr. Jerilynn Prior made a detailed study of 66 women who were not ovulating but who were having regular periods. They were losing 2 percent of their bone mass every year and had low progesterone levels. Dr. Prior found she could reverse the bone loss by giving 10 mg of Provera daily. She believes that the hormone progesterone is very important for bone health. She also advises women to find out if they are ovulating because a woman who is not ovulating regularly has a higher risk of bone loss. However, a new study involving young women taking injectable medroxyprogesterone acetate (Depo-Provera), synthetic progesterone for birth control, found that their bone density was 7 percent lower than that of young women not using the drug.

Dr. Prior used progestins in her studies, and there is much confusion between these progestins and natural progesterone. Natural progesterone is synthesized in a laboratory from the wild yam or from soy. It is what is known as a "bioidentical" hormone because its molecular structure is identical to a woman's own hormone progesterone produced by her ovaries. Its structure is completely different from synthetic progesterone whose proper name is progestin. Progestin is often mistakenly called progesterone and confused with natural progesterone.

The Popularity of Progesterone

The popularity of progesterone is based largely on the work and the writing of Dr. John Lee, an internationally recognized authority on fluoride and a clinical instructor at the University of California Medical School. He is the author of the book, *What Your Doctor May Not Tell You About Menopause*. Dr. Lee believed that applying progesterone to the skin in the form of a cream helped increase bone mineral density in postmenopausal women. In his small study, 100 women used the cream during a three-year period. Sixty-three of the women had bone density tests that indicated an average bone density increase of 15.4 percent over the three-year period, compared with an expected loss of 4.5 percent. Most of the women studied had previously fractured bones, but no new fractures were reported during the three-year study. This study was conducted as an observational study—that is, there was no control group and, as such, was viewed with skepticism by the medical community.

In addition to the progesterone, the women in the study were encouraged to consume green, leafy vegetables; to avoid cigarettes and carbonated beverages; to supplement with calcium, vitamin D3, non-acidic vitamin C, and the many bone-building cofactors; and to participate in a regular exercise program. Some of the women were also taking estrogen vaginal cream. Because each of these additional recommendations may have a positive influence on bone density, it is difficult to say whether it was the progesterone or the combination of the strategies that had the effect.

In a more recent, randomized controlled trial in the United States, 102 healthy postmenopausal women used progesterone cream and calcium and vitamin supplements. During the one-year study, there was no significant difference in bone density between the progesterone and the control groups. However, the natural progesterone was effective in relieving menopausal symptoms. It may be possible that the effect of natural progesterone on bone may not become apparent until after more than one year of use, or it may require higher dosages. Another study showed that transdermal progesterone was effective in raising blood levels of natural progesterone.

Natural progesterone is very safe and appears to have few side effects. Personally, I believe that bioidentical natural progesterone in the form of creams or prescription pills (known as Prometrium) can have a beneficial effect on bone to help prevent bone loss and to treat osteopenia, but only as a part of a comprehensive program that includes exercise and supplements.

In my experience, natural progesterone alone is not enough to build bone once osteoporosis has occurred. I prescribe natural progesterone (alone or in combination with bioidentical estrogen and testosterone, and bisphos-phonate medications if necessary), always in addition to exercise and a comprehensive food-based, bone-building supplement to treat osteoporosis once it has occurred.

Testosterone

Testosterone is a hormone that is important to bone health, particularly for men, but it can also be useful for women. There is a lot of exciting research going on in this field. Studies so far indicate that testosterone in the form of transdermal creams and pills can help reverse bone loss in men. This is a very promising research area. Even now, natural testosterone can be safely added to treatment regimens for both men and postmenopausal women whose free testosterone levels (the amount of active testosterone in the bloodstream) are low.

NON-DRUG TREATMENTS FOR OSTEOPOROSIS

Dynamic Motion Therapy

An exciting new treatment will be used by NASA to help prevent bone loss on the International Space Center, known as dynamic motion therapy (DMT). DMT consists of a small device the size of a bathroom scale. This device vibrates the person who steps on it using high frequency low intensity vibrations, it stimulates bones in the same way that muscles did when we were younger. Standing on this gently vibrating device for 20 minutes, five times a week has been shown to promote a yearly increase in bone density by an average of one to two per cent in the studies conducted so far. It may be useful not only for women and men with low bone density who can't use drugs, but also for teenagers and children with cerebral palsy.

Health Canada has licenced it as a class II medical device, allowing it to be sold nationwide in Canada. Check the website www.juvent.com to find out how to order this device. This and other non-drug approaches are fully explored in Renée Newman's insightful and helpful book *Osteoporosis Prevention*.

Good Balance and Core Strength Can Prevent Falling

Osteoporosis can make bones vulnerable—falls can break them. Almost 90 percent of osteoporosis-related hip fractures, and more than 90 percent of pelvic and hipbone fractures, and 50 percent of spinal fractures result from falls.

Good balance depends on your vision. Therefore, do some walking or balancing exercises each day with your eyes closed to train your brain to keep you upright and steady. People who are physically fit and active have better balance and far fewer bone fracturing falls in their later years. Have your vision and hearing tested annually.

Fall-prevention techniques may be better than medications at reducing the death rate from hip fracture. Research shows that a fall to the side, as opposed to forward or backward falls, increases the risk of hip fracture by about six times, and is considered a much greater risk than lower bone density for hip fracture.

Mary Tinetti, M.D., of Yale University, took a group of 300 women and men aged 70 or older. Half the group, the control group, received no special care. The other half learned exercises to improve their strength, balance, and coordination, which resulted in 48 percent fewer falls—a significant reduction for a group at such high risk.

Western medical researchers are beginning to appreciate what Eastern medical researchers have known for many years—that Tai Chi, Qigong, and hatha yoga can dramatically improve your balance. Poor balance is not only a concern for us in our senior years; we are all vulnerable to falls.

It is estimated that 50–60 percent of falls happen in the home and 85 percent of those are caused by common "domestic hazards" like throw rugs, extension cords, slippery floors, dim lights, or clutter on the floor. Give your home a serious safety check-up and immediately correct any problems you find.

Follow the core-strengthening program in Chapter 9, "Ramp Up Bone-Building Metabolic Exercise," to feel more secure and steady on your feet, improve your muscle and bone strength, enhance balance, and significantly increase your fluid range of motion for a lifetime.

WHAT DOES THIS HAVE TO DO WITH YOU?

What should be clear to you by now is that if you have been diagnosed with osteoporosis or osteopenia, there is a lot you can do to treat and even reverse your condition naturally. Remember that drugs can be, if needed, an addition to any successful treatment, but not a substitute for a healthy lifestyle that combines exercise, bone-building foods, and a bone-building supplement. For each individual, the optimal program will vary a little to meet his or her biological individuality.

The future looks bright. I'm convinced that within the next four or five years, we will see major breakthroughs in the development of medications and treatments to help us keep our bones strong and healthy.

In the meantime, though, it is important to eat well, exercise often, get a BMD and both blood and urine tests if you are at high risk. If you have a problem, start treating it right away with a natural, food-based, "molecular-targeted" bone-building supplement and, if necessary, with one of the many osteoporosis drugs available.

About 10 years ago I became intrigued by the bone-building process. I had a bone scan and was diagnosed with osteopenia. When the radiologist gave me the diagnosis, I felt very frightened. I became motivated to build up my bone mineral density and strength naturally. I followed the step-by-step sensible action plan and comprehensive bone-building program that nutritional and lifestyle researcher Sam Graci has set out in this book. I have opted not to use medications, and my bone density has greatly improved—I no longer have osteopenia. But the biggest benefit has been increased levels of overall health, vitality, and self-confidence. I believe that the majority of you can achieve the same increased bone density and health I have by simply following the breakthrough and unique action plan for every decade of your life found in Chapter 10 of this book.

You too will see and feel the amazing results I did as you solve your personal bone-building equation. Metaphorically, our bones are comparable to a foundation of a house. When we go back to basics and strengthen the foundation, we are ensuring that our house will stand for a long time. Each new day will be filled with a renewed appreciation for your revitalized bone health, well-being, and vitality.

Let a vibrant, balanced, and healthy physical, mental, emotional, and spiritual life be the rallying cry of a new generation of motivated men and women who commit to optimizing and maintaining the absolute magic of their healthy bones, joints, brain, body, and spirit. Medical research breakthroughs can light the pathway to our ultimate well-being. Walking it is still up to us.

As Sam would say, "Healthy bones, healthy brain, healthy heart, healthy life, healthy you!"

Part III

A Research Scientist's Perspective on Bone-Building

Written by: Dr. Leticia Rao, Ph.D., Director of the Calcium Research Lab, St. Michael's Hospital, University of Toronto, Faculty of Medicine

CHAPTER 13

Clinical Breakthroughs in Bone-Building Research

A NATURAL PRESCRIPTION FOR SUPERIOR BONE-BUILDING

Introduction: Oxidative Stress: The Problem

In various chapters in this book, Sam Graci has touched upon the detrimental effects of oxidative stress caused by reactive oxygen species (ROS) to our health and well-being. There is also now ample evidence to suggest that oxidative stress is associated with the pathogenesis of bone loss. Considering the possible adverse side effects of the conventional system of medicine in the management of age-related bone loss, there is an increasing demand for the use of natural components of foods for the prevention and treatment of this debilitating ailment that also constricts your fluid biomechanical movements.

Government advisory panels have strongly suggested that we consume five to 10 servings of fresh fruit and vegetables each day. As a clinical bone researcher, I have focused on the various natural pigments that a plant uses to defend itself from ultraviolet radiation, bacteria, viruses, fungus, and to act as natural antioxidants to prevent oxidative stress and free radical damage. Scientists now acknowledge that more than 60 human diseases such as cancer, heart disease, diabetes, Alzheimer's, and osteoporosis evolve to some extent because of oxidative stress and free radical damage (see Figure 13-1). We have estimated that there are 10,000 different phytonutrients (*phyto*, meaning from plants). There are 8,000 of these phytonutrients that act as antioxidants in the human body, and can be classified into two primary groups: polyphenols and carotenoids, which give plants their diversity of colors. I would like to focus on the clinical research I have completed and give examples of one polyphenol and one carotenoid and the positive effect they may have on promoting superior bone-building for a lifetime. In this chapter, I will review recent *in vitro* and *in vivo* research studies, including ours, which shed light into how the antioxidants lycopene and polyphenols may lower the risk of porous, weak bones, and osteoporosis.

Bone Cells and Bone in Osteoporosis: The Victims

Bone is a dynamic tissue as it is continuously renewed throughout life by bone remodeling, which involves the coupled events of the removal of old bone by osteoclast cells and the building of new bone by osteoblast cells (1). These two types of cells are the major bone cells involved in the prevention of osteoporosis through their interaction with multiple molecular agents, including hormones, growth factors, and cytokines during the remodeling process. It is also now clear that free radical assaults on bone-building cells cause acute inflammation and biochemical chaos that leads to rapid bone-breakdown.

Osteoporosis, one of a number of metabolic bone diseases that result from a disturbance of the bone remodeling process (1), is characterized by low bone mass and micro-architectural deterioration of bone tissue, causing increased bone fragility and greater risk of fracture (2). It occurs predominantly among women over the age of 45 because of their loss of estrogen at menopause (3) and also among men over the age of 55 with their low levels of the sex hormone testosterone (4). Known as the "silent epidemic," it may affect one in two women and one in four men over the age of 50 to some degree. In bone loss, the remodeling process becomes significantly more active than the normal process with a primary increase in bone resorption or breakdown and a counterbalancing but insufficient increase in bone formation (5). The early manifestation of the risk of osteoporosis in men and women is an increase in both bone turnover markers of resorption and formation (3). Bone turnover markers have therefore become measurement parameters to predict risk of fractures among men and women (6). We have used the bone turnover markers in our clinical study to evaluate the role of lycopene, a natural component of tomatoes, and polyphenols, the colorful phytonutrients in produce.

CLINICAL BREAKTHROUGH NUMBER 1

Polyphenols: The Water-Soluble Antioxidant Solution

Polyphenols, the water-soluble plant pigments, are a group of plant chemical substances that have more than one phenol group per molecule. The polyphenols, which are responsible for the coloring of some plants and their antioxidant properties, have potential health benefits, including the prevention of cardiovascular diseases, cancers, neurodegenerative diseases, diabetes, and osteoporosis. Sam Graci has written a comprehensive review of polyphenols in chapters 5, 6, and 10, with emphasis on food sources and their beneficial effects on bone. In the latter part of this chapter, I will discuss our study on the effects of polyphenols on the bone-building cells, the osteoblasts.

Other sources of polyphenol antioxidants include fruit, vegetables, red wine, green tea, and the traditional Mediterranean diet. A growing body of research shows that the polyphenols in green tea, especially epigallocatechin gallate (EGCG) can assist in the reduction of both inflammation and free radical proliferation in bone-building cells. I recommend that you consume 2 or 3 cups of green tea per day, each of which will provide approximately 90 mg of EGCG. The highest grade of green tea is Japanese matcha, made of the finest green tea leaves.

(There is some concern from recent experimental studies that green tea may induce a deficiency of the B vitamin folic acid by its inhibition of an enzyme involved in folate metabolism. Therefore, if you are drinking more than 2 cups of green tea a day, then taking 400 mcg of folic acid daily in a bone-building supplement is advisable, especially if you are pregnant, intending to become pregnant, or if you are lactating.)

Research Studies on the Role of Polyphenols in Bone Health

Polyphenols and Bone-Building

Ines Urquiaga and Federico Leighton, of Pontificia Universidad Católica de Chile, stated in a review article that the health benefits associated with fruits, vegetables, red wine, tea, and Mediterranean diets are probably linked to the polyphenol antioxidants they contain (7). Studies on animals or cultured human cell lines support a role of polyphenols in the prevention of cardiovascular diseases, cancers, neurodegenerative diseases, diabetes, and osteoporosis. The most commonly studied polyphenol is epigallocatechin-3-Gallate (EGCG), the most abundant polyphenol in green tea. Indeed, epidemiological studies show a positive association between tea drinking—including green tea—and bone mineral density (8). EGCG, the polyphenol from green tea, has been shown to inhibit the expression of matrix metalloproteinase 9 (MMP-9) in osteoblasts and the formation of osteoclasts, which suggests that EGCG may prevent the alveolar bone resorption that occurs in periodontal diseases (9). H_2O_2-induced alterations of osteoblast viability and reduction in alkaline phosphatase activity were prevented by pre-incubating the osteoblasts with green tea polyphenol (10). The polyphenol Phloridzin (Phlo), a flavonoid in apple, was found to provide protection against ovariectomy-induced osteopenia (11).

We have studied the role of polyphenols on the ability of osteoblasts to form bone. For this purpose, we used the "green drink" greens+ nutritional supplement, a blend of several botanical products, because it is a rich source of polyphenols. To study the effects of greens+ on differentiation and bone formation in human osteoblasts, the osteoblast-like SaOS-2 cells were grown in medium that supports bone formation in the presence or absence of the polyphenolic extract of greens+.

The most important finding of this study is that the water-soluble component containing polyphenols from greens+ increased proliferation of human osteoblasts at early time points of addition. Furthermore, it stimulated the alkaline phosphatase (ALP) activity when added at early time points at lower concentrations and inhibited it at later time points at higher concentrations. Continuous addition of a water-soluble component containing polyphenols from *greens+* showed a dose and time-dependent stimulation of bone nodule formation. Our results showed that *greens+* extract influenced human osteoblasts in a manner consistent with its effects on subsequent differentiation of osteoprogenitors toward progression to a bone-forming stage.

A comparison of the effects of *greens+* extract with those of standard epicatechin, a major polyphenolic component of green tea, showed that *greens+* was more effective than epicatechin. This may be explained by the fact that *greens+* extract contains a mixture of polyphenols, including quercetin (177.25 µg/g), apigenin (133.31µg/g), kaempferol (98.56µg/g), and luteolin (58.28µg/g) (Rao, A.V., personal communication), and that the greater potency observed for *greens+* may be a result of the synergistic effects of the different polyphenols (12).

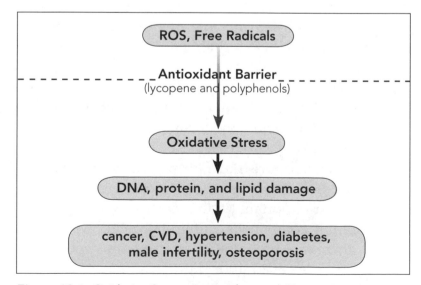

Figure 13-1: Oxidative Stress, Antioxidant and Chronic Diseases

Recent observation from our laboratory showed that *greens+* extract added under the same conditions as those used in this present study inhibited the intracellular reactive oxygen species production in SaOS-2 cells (13). These findings suggest that the polyphenols present in the *greens+* extract act through their antioxidant properties (13).

A nutritional supplement called *greens+bone builder* has recently been formulated and contains, in addition to the basic *greens+*, other food components that have been clinically shown to be beneficial to bone-building. These components include antioxidants, vitamins, minerals, trace minerals, and amino acids. The role of each of these components in the prevention of osteoporosis is not completely clear at the present time. We plan to investigate *in vitro*, using our mineralizing cell culture system, whether the additional supplements will have a more potent effect than the *greens+* alone. We also plan to carry out a clinical study to determine whether intervention with *greens+bone builder* in postmenopausal women with high bone turnover markers will reduce oxidative stress and bone turnover markers and improve their antioxidant status, thus decreasing their risk for osteoporosis.

CLINICAL BREAKTHROUGH NUMBER 2

Lycopene: The Lipid-Soluble Antioxidant Solution

Lycopene belongs to the family of carotenoid compounds in fruits and vegetables. They are synthesized by plants and microorganisms, but not by animals and humans. Hence, whatever lycopene we have in our bodies is accumulated through the food we eat. Lycopene is the pigment that gives tomatoes their red color, and is one of four main carotenoids normally found in human blood and tissue. Although red-colored fruits and vegetables are the most common sources of dietary lycopene, not all red-colored plants contain lycopene. North Americans obtain 85 percent of their dietary lycopene from tomatoes and processed tomato products. There is about 5 mg of lycopene per 100 gm of ripe tomato fruit (equivalent to one medium tomato). Lycopene concentration in tomatoes increases significantly during the ripening process. Green and yellow tomatoes do not contain lycopene. Other sources of lycopene are watermelon, pink guavas, and pink grapefruit (14). However, the lycopene content of these fruits are much lower than the amount present in tomatoes and tomato products.

The health benefit from lycopene may result from its ability to scavenge singlet-oxygen, bestowing it a potent antioxidant property (15). However, other mechanisms such as effects on gap junctions (16) and cell cycling (17) have been reported and need to be tested further.

Lycopene is absorbed more efficiently from processed tomato products than the raw tomatoes because of its conversion with heat processing from the all-trans to its cis-isomeric configuration. Since lycopene is a lipid-soluble compound that is absorbed through a chylomicron-mediated mechanism, the presence of small amounts of lipids will further enhance its absorption (18).

The reported average daily intake levels of lycopene vary considerably from 0.7 mg per day in Finland to 25 mg per day in Canada. According to Dr. Venket Rao, there is no official recommended daily intake of lycopene, but based on published research, an intake of 7 mg of lycopene per day is suggested. Lower blood levels of lycopene are associated with higher body weight, aging, smoking, and increased risk of health disorders.

Evidence that lycopene has a role in the prevention of chronic diseases has been very well documented by epidemiological, tissue culture, and animal studies. Human intervention studies are now being conducted to validate epidemiological observations and to understand the mechanisms of action of lycopene in disease prevention. Osteoporosis is the only chronic disease that has not been studied thoroughly. Our laboratory is actively carrying out *in vitro* and *in vivo* research on the role of lycopene in bone health, which we will review below.

Research on the Role of Lycopene in Bone Health

There is now convincing evidence of a role for lycopene in osteoporosis. The evidence is based on lycopene's potent antioxidant properties; the well-known role of oxidative stress in osteoporosis and the bone cells involved in the pathogenesis of osteoporosis; the studies on the effects of lycopene in these cells in culture, and, more recently, the results of a study on lycopene intake and bone resorption markers in postmenopausal women. Although oxidative stress has been associated with osteoporosis and the activity and function of osteoblasts and osteoclasts, the cellular and molecular mechanisms of their actions and the role played by lycopene are not completely clear at the present time. In this section, we will review the evidence for the role of lycopene in osteoblasts and osteoclasts and our ongoing clinical study, which is the first study to evaluate lycopene from a nutritional supplement and tomato juice in the prevention of osteoporosis in postmenopausal women.

Lycopene and Bone Cells

Effects of Lycopene on Osteoclasts: In order to explore the hypothesis that lycopene can inhibit mineral resorption, osteoclast formation, and the production of ROS, Leticia Rao and colleague (19) cultured cells from bone marrow prepared from rat femur into 16-well calcium phosphate-coated Osteologic™ Multi-test Slides in a medium supplemented with dexamethasone, ß-glycerophosphate, and ascorbic acid. The cells were treated with varying doses of lycopene in the absence or presence of the bone-resorbing agent parathyroid hormone [PTH-(1–34)] at the start of culture and at each medium change (i.e., every 48 hours). On day eight, mineral resorption pits were quantified. Similar, parallel experiments were carried out in 12-well plastic dishes to assess tartrate-resistant acid phosphatase (TRAP) activity. Results revealed that lycopene inhibited the mineral resorption by osteoclasts, and that the inhibition was greater in the presence of more concentrated lycopene. The number of cells that were stained with the NBT reduction product formazan were decreased by treatment with 10^{-5} M lycopene indicating that lycopene inhibited the formation of ROS-secreting osteoclasts. Rao et al. concluded that lycopene inhibited basal and PTH-stimulated osteoclastic mineral resorption and formation of TRAP+ multinucleated osteoclasts, as well as the ROS produced by osteoclasts. These findings are new and may be important in the pathogenesis, treatment, and prevention of osteoporosis.

Ishimi et al. also reported the effect of lycopene on osteoclast formation and bone resorption using murine osteoclasts formed in co-culture with calvarial osteoblasts (20). Their results differed from those of Rao et al.

(19) in that they found that lycopene inhibited the PTH-induced, but not the basal, TRAP+ multinucleated cell formation. Furthermore, they could not demonstrate any effect of lycopene on bone resorption. They also did not study the effect of lycopene on ROS production. The difference in the results from the two laboratories may be related to the species of cells used.

Effects of Lycopene on Osteoblasts: The studies on the effects of lycopene on osteoblasts are limited to two reports (21, 22). Kim et al. (22) reported that lycopene had a stimulatory effect on ALP activity, a marker of osteoblastic differentiation in more mature cells. However, depending on the time of addition, lycopene had an inhibitory or no effect on younger SaOS-Dex cells. These findings were the first report on the effect of lycopene on human osteoblasts. In another study Park et al. (21) reported that ALP activity was stimulated in the mouse cell line MC3T3. Both studies reported that ALP activity was stimulated by lycopene.

Clinical Studies on the Role of Lycopene in Postmenopausal Women

In order to show the association of lycopene with post-menopausal osteoporosis, a cross-sectional study was conducted in which 33 postmenopausal women aged 50–60 years provided seven-day dietary records and blood samples (23). The participant population was confined to this age group since postmenopause is associated with a global increase in bone turnover markers (24, 25) that predict bone loss and osteoporosis in post-menopausal women (5); this increase is generally more prominent after one year of menopause and shown to increase until age 60. Thus, one of the objectives of our current clinical study at St. Michael's Hospital is to test whether the serum lycopene correlates inversely with the oxidative stress parameters, lipid peroxidation and protein thiols, and the bone turnover markers ALP activity (bone formation) and cross-linked N-telopeptides of type I collagen (NTx) (bone resorption). Total antioxidant capacity and serum lycopene were also measured from serum samples.

The participants were grouped into quartiles according to their serum lycopene per kilogram body weight (nM/kg) and correlation analyses were carried out using the Newman-Keuls post test. The most important and interesting findings to date are the significant decreases in protein oxidation as indicated by increased thiols ($p<0.05$) and decreased NTx values ($p<0.005$) as levels of serum lycopene increase (23). Since there was a significant positive correlation between serum lycopene levels and dietary lycopene intake as determined from the estimated food records ($p<0.01$), our results support the hypothesis that dietary lycopene acts as an effective antioxidant, reducing oxidative stress and bone turnover markers. Our observations suggest an important role for lycopene mediated via its antioxidant property in reducing the risk of osteoporosis. Dietary intervention studies with varying doses and sources of lycopene are currently being conducted to determine the beneficial effects of lycopene in the prevention and management of osteoporosis. Participants are randomly assigned to one of the following four supplement groups: 15 mg lycopene group consuming regular tomato juice from Heinz, Canada; 35 mg lycopene group consuming lycopene-enriched tomato juice from Kagome, Japan; 15 mg and lycopene capsule group or placebo capsule group, both from LycoRed, Israel. Following a one-month washout period, participants consume their supplement twice daily and give fasting blood samples and seven-day dietary records at the beginning and after two and four months of consumption. Measurement parameters are similar to those of the cross-sectional study described above. This study is ongoing and is the first to evaluate lycopene in the prevention of osteoporosis in postmenopausal women.

Although it is too early to suggest that eating tomatoes and tomato products will prevent osteoporosis, it would be a healthy practice to include tomatoes and tomato products in the diet as a source of lycopene for the prevention of oxidative stress-related chronic diseases,including osteoporosis. The final results of our study may indicate that lycopene may be used either as adietary alternative to drug therapy or as a complement to the drugs used by men and women at risk for osteoporosis.

CONCLUDING REMARKS

It is now evident that natural colorful components in fruit and vegetables are good for optimum bone-repair and bone-building. Examples of these are the antioxidants lipid-soluble lycopene and the water-soluble polyphenols. These antioxidants are now being incorporated into biocompatible, food-based, bone-building supplements. Therefore, the use of a comprehensive bone-building supplement may be required to achieve optimum bone health and may be a good alternative, combined with wise lifestyle choices, for the prevention of osteoporosis.

Product Resources

A "MOLECULAR-TARGETED," FOOD-BASED BONE-BUILDING SUPPLEMENT

Not all concentrated food-based bone-building supplements are of the same high quality. *greens+* is the only clinically proven bone-building formula, tested by the University of Toronto Medical School and *greens+* by the School of Pharmacology, that proved to boost energy, antioxidant levels, alkalinity, and increase bone-building. *greens+* has won a gold medal on many occasions in both Canada and the United States from the Canadian Health Food Association, National Nutritional Foods Association as "Product of the Year" in the U.S., and The Inventors Club of America, Inc.'s prestigious International Hall of Fame award for exceptional quality.

In Canada
greens+
greens+ bone builder
greens+ daily detox
greens+ extra energy
greens+ kids
greens+ multi+

meno herbal support for women
rolls of pH paper for urine and saliva testing are available from:

Genuine Health
Toronto, Ontario
Toll-free: (877) 500-7888
Website: www.genuinehealth.com

In the United States
Life Extension *Herbal Mix* is available from:
Life Extension
Ft. Lauderdale, Florida
Toll-free: (800) 544-4440
Website: www.lef.org

greens+ is available from:
Orange Peel Enterprises, Inc.
Vero Beach, Florida
Toll-free: (800) 643-1210
Website: www.greensplus.com

LONG-CHAIN OMEGA-3 ESSENTIAL FATTY ACID FISH OILS RICH IN "MOOD-SMART" EPA AND "BONE-SMART" DHA

Following the brilliant research of omega-3 fatty acid researchers such as Dr. Artemis P. Simopoulos, president of The Center for Genetics; Dr. Joseph Hibbelin, of the National Institutes of Health; Dr. Zanarini, of Harvard Medical School; Dr. Bruce J. Holub, of the University of Guelph; and Dr. Alan Logan, director of CAM Research Consulting in New York, Genuine Health has formulated and developed the id System™ enteric-coated *o3mega* wild fish oil formulations to therapeutically help with specific conditions. These pharmaceutical-grade fish oils are either steamed or molecularly distilled, and are third-party tested for potency and purity by the renowned Nutrasource Diagnostics IFOS System at the University of Guelph.

In Canada and the United States
Genuine Health, Toronto, Ontario, Canada
Toll-free: (877) 500-7888
Website: www.genuinehealth.com

Life Extension, Ft. Lauderdale, Florida, U.S.
Toll-free: (800) 544-4440
Website: www.lef.org

1. *o3mega*: 180 mg EPA and 120 mg DHA per softgel for general use

2. *o3mega extra strength*: 400 mg EPA and 200 mg DHA for maximum benefits of omega-3

3. *o3mega+ pump*: 105 mg EPA, 69 mg DHA, and 88 mg GLA from borage oil per softgel for a healthy cardiovascular system provides the exact 4:2 ratio of EPA/DHA:GLA used in research for heart health

4. *o3mega+ fit*: 146 mg EPA, 96 mg DHA, and 49 mg GLA from borage oil per softgel for those exercising or on a diet because both lose EPA and DHA reserves quickly

5. *o3mega+ think*: 100 mg EPA and 250 mg DHA per softgel for a bright, alert boost in brainpower, cognitive function, and maintenance of your eyes and nerves

6. *o3mega+ joy*: 500 mg EPA and 25 mg DHA per soft-gel for enhanced, superior, improved mood and well-being; scientific studies prove EPA regulates depression

7. *o3mega+ glow*: 250 mg EPA, 75 mg red tomato extract, 50 mg ascorbyl palmitate (fat-soluble vitamin C), 25 IU vitamin E, 25 mg bilberry complex

8. *o3mega+ 3679*: 108 mg EPA, 72 mg DHA, plus healthy omega-6, -7, and -9 from 300 mg borage oil and 200 mg macadamia nut oil for an updated and complete version of the popular omega-3, -6, -9 supplements

9. *Super EPA/DHA*: with sesame lignans and olive extract, 1,400 mg of EPA, 1,000 mg of DHA, 530 mg olive fruit extract, and 20 mg of sesame lignans in four capsules

Note: #1, 5, 6, and 8 are also available in a naturally flavored, liquid format.

Please note: *o3mega+ 3679* is the bone-building formula I would prefer that you use in either the traditional softgel form, or in a naturally flavored liquid format.

Suggested Supplements

In Canada and the United States

- *abs+*: CLA and EGCG from green tea; both proven in clinical trials to enhance significant abdominal fat reduction and weight loss safely and naturally: www.genuinehealth.com

	In Canada	In The United States
Bone-Restore	**Life Extension** *Bone-Restore* provides a potent source of calcium along with super-critical micro-nutrients for bone-building, a superior calcium-absorption formula. Toll-free: (800) 544-4440 Website: www.lef.org	**Life Extension** *Bone-Restore* provides a potent source of calcium along with super-critical micro-nutrients for bone-building, a superior calcium-absorption formula. Toll-free: (800) 544-4440 Website: www.lef.org
Borage Oil, Black Currant Oil	**Omega Nutrition Canada Inc.** Toll-free: (800) 661-3529 Website: www.omegaflo.com	**Omega Nutrition U.S.A. Inc.** Toll-free: (800) 661-3529 Website: www.omegaflo.com
DME™ Extra Virgin Coconut Oil	**Alpha Health Products** Toll-free: (800) 663-2212 Website: www.alphahealth.ca	**Alpha Health Products** Toll-free: (800) 663-2212 Website: www.alphahealth.ca
Evening Primrose Oil	**Efamol** Toll-free: (888) 318-5222 Website: www.efamol.com	**Efamol** Toll-free: (888) 318-5222 Website: www.efamol.com
High-Alpha 100 Percent Whey Isolate Protein Powder	***proteins+*** Genuine Health Toll-free: (877) 500-7888 Website: www.genuinehealth.com	***Enhanced Life Extension Protein*** Life Extension Toll-free: (800) 544-4440 Website: www.lef.org
Seabuckthorn Omega-7	**Seabuckthorn International Inc.** Toll-free: (877) 767-6101 Website: www.seabuckthorn.com	**Seabuckthorn International Inc.** Toll-free: (877) 767-6101 Website: www.seabuckthorn.com

- Life Extension *Herbal Mix*: pharmaceutical-grade super-absorbable CoQ10, resveratrol, COGNITEX a neuroprotection complex, pharmaceutical-grade bioidentical DHEA and sublingual melatonin, vitamin E as tocopherols and tocotrienols: www.lef.org or (800) 544-4440

- *greens+ multi+*, award-winning food-based multivitamin/mineral: www.genuinehealth.com

- *Bio-K+*, living probiotic cultures, preferred source, fermented yogurt medium, with 50 billion viable, active bacteria per 3.5 oz container: www.biokplus.com

- Probiotics, enteric-coated—Jarrow-EPS: www.jarrow.com and Flora www.florahealth.com

- Maca powder (organic gelatinized) for power, balance, and vitality—Navitas naturals: www.navitasnaturals.com

- Olive oil: five-star, organic, cold-pressed, extra-virgin olive oil. In Canada, contact: Biolea at www.rawthyme@yahoo.ca; and in the United States, contact: Soler Romero at www.odysseyfoods.com

- Migraines, SISU *Petadolex*® butterbur extract: www.petadolex.ca

- Joint and muscle pain, *Atrosan gel*, fresh arnica gel: www.bioforce.ca

- NEEDAK® soft-bounce Rebounders: in Canada (877) 988-9300 or in the U.S. (800) 334-2605

- pH water machines, the Regency II: www.kabencompany.com or (866) 522-3626

10 EXCELLENT NEWSLETTERS TO KEEP YOU UPDATED

1. *Health and Happiness Newsletter*, free: www.genuinehealth.com

2. *Life Extension Magazine* (monthly): (800) 544-4440; cost $75.00 U.S. for annual membership, magazine, and product discounts. An outstanding website! www.lef.org

3. *National Institutes of Health* (NIH), free: www.nih.gov

4. *Seafood Safety*: www.ifosprogram.com

5. *Berkeley Wellness Newsletter*: www.berkeleywellness.com

6. *Harvard Health Letter* and *Harvard Women's Health Watch*: www.health.harvard.edu

7. *Townsend Letter for Doctors and Patients*: www.townsend.com

8. *Tufts University Health and Nutrition Letter*: www.healthletter.tufts.edu

9. *National Osteoporosis Foundation (NOF)*: www.nof.org

10. *International Osteoporosis Foundation (IOF)*: www.osteofound.org

BIOIDENTICAL HORMONE RESTORATIVE THERAPY

Please look at the Life Extension Foundation website www.lef.org to view the ideal bloodstream range of hormones and biomarkers of aging recommended for your age. If you are 40 or older, please look at the information on melatonin and DHEA or review Chapter 3 of this book.

Take the recommended blood tests, along with the ideal range you should be in for each blood test, to a knowledgeable physician who uses natural, bioidentical hormone restorative therapy. Hormone restoration of DHEA, melatonin, estrogen, progesterone, free testosterone, DHT, etc., must be based on your personal, comprehensive blood tests and custom designed to your particular need, age, and level of well-being.

A compounding pharmacist will make a superabsorbable transdermal cream that you simply rub inside your thighs or arms to restore balance and a more youthful hormone equilibrium.

Furthermore, contact Life Extension Foundation for a list of physicians and medical clinics across North America who are up to date and familiar with hormone restorative therapy. Their medical advisory board is simply superlative. The following chart illustrates their reference ranges.

In many cases, a "Standard Reference Range" reflects what is expected in the average population. Since cancer and cardiovascular disease remain the number one killers of North Americans, you don't ever want to be part of the "average" range when it comes to cardiovascular disease or cancer risk factors.

By keeping your blood levels in the "Optimal Range," rather than the average "Standard Reference Range," you take advantage of the increasing volume of evidence showing that many cancers, heart attacks, and strokes are preventable.

As you can see, the "Standard Reference Range" often dangerously differs from what the published research indicates is protective against cardiovascular disease.

Blood Test	What the "Standard Reference Range" Allows	The "Optimal" Level Where YOU Want to Be
Fibrinogen	Up to 460 mg/dL	Under 300 mg/dL
C-reactive protein	Up to 4.9 mg/L	Under 2 mg/L Some studies indicate C-reactive protein levels should be below 1.3 mg/L
Homocysteine	Up to 15 micro mol/L	Under 7 micro mol/L
Glucose	Up to 109 mg/dL	Under 100 mg/dL
Iron	Up to 180 mg/dL	Under 100 mcg/dL
Cholesterol	Up to 199 mg/dL *	Between 180-220 mg/dL
LDL cholesterol	Up to 129 mg/dL	Under 100 mg/dL
HDL cholesterol	No lower than 35 mg/dL	Over 50 mg/dL
Triglycerides	Up to 199 mg/dL	Under 100 mg/dL
DHEA	Males: No lower than 80 mcg/dL Females: No lower than 35 mcg/dL	Between 400–560 mcg/dL Between 350–430 mcg/dL

*There are numerous published studies indicating that cholesterol levels should ideally be under 200 mg/dL. The Life Extension Foundation believes it is more important to concentrate on suppressing dangerous LDL cholesterol and increasing beneficial HDL levels. If other risk factors such as homocysteine, fibrinogen, C-reactive protein, etc., are individually adjusted to reflect "optimal" ranges, then a slightly higher total cholesterol of up to 220 might be acceptable. Please note that cholesterol levels below 180 mg/dL present increased risk of hemorrhagic stroke and other diseases, so it is important that people maintain a minimal amount of cholesterol, i.e., 180 mg/dL of blood. It is important to note that in the past, cholesterol levels well above 200 were considered within the "normal" reference range.

Please note: Because cholesterol is a precursor, or building block, for many hormones, "cholesterol deficiency" may lead to diminished production of basic hormones. In 2002, the journal *Neuropsychobiology* and the *American Journal of Medical Science* clearly correlated low total cholesterol with mental illness.

Hormone tests may become unique biomarkers in assessing behavioral and psychiatric disorders in children, adolescents, and adults. By finding safer solutions to balancing hormones as a first step, many ADD and ADHD conditions may be able to avoid prescription drugs.

Female Hormone Profile		
Hormone Blood Test	**"Standard Reference Range"**	**"Optimal" Level**
DHEA-S	30–700 mcg/dL	150–350 mcg/dL
Cortisol	5–29 mcg/dL	9–14 mcg/dL
Estrogen	30–480 pg/mL	180–200 pg/mL (women under 50)
		60–120 pg/mL (women over 50)
Progesterone	300–26,000 pg/mL	2,000–14,000 pg/mL (women under 50)
		2,000–8,000 pg/mL (women over 50)
Total testosterone	140–760 pg/mL	120–900 pg/mL
TSH	0.2–5.5 mU/L	1.0–2.0 mU/L
Free T3	2.60–4.80 pg/mL	2.80–3.20 pg/mL
Free T4	0.70–1.53 ng/dL	1.2–1.4 ng/dL
Total T3	60–181 ng/dL	120–124 ng/dL
Total T4	4.5–12.0 mcg/dL	7.5–8.1 mcg/dL

Male Hormone Profile		
Hormone Blood Test	"Standard Reference Range"	"Optimal" Level
DHEA-S	20–620 mcg/dL	250–450 mcg/dL
Cortisol	5–29 mcg/dL	9–14 mcg/dL
Total estrogens	40–115 pg/mL	Less than 100 pg/mL
Estradiol	21–50 pg/mL	Less than 40 pg/mL
Progesterone	300–1,200 pg/mL	1,500–2,500 pg/mL
Total testosterone	2,700–9,700 pg/mL	6,000–9,000 pg/mL
TSH	0.2–5.5 mU/L	1.0–2.0 mU/L
Free T3	2.60–4.80 pg/mL	2.90–3.20 pg/mL
Free T4	0.70–1.53 ng/dL	1.2–1.4 ng/dL
IGF-1	114–492 ng/mL	200–300 ng/mL

WELLNESS RESOURCES

The following alphabetical resource listings have websites and telephone numbers for current health information, self-study courses, research results, or to locate a health practitioner.

Alive Academy of Nutrition health advisor self-study: www.alive.com or (800) 663-6580

American Academy of Anti-Aging Medicine: www.worldhealth.net

American Association of Naturopathic Physicians: www.naturopathic.org or (877) 969-2267

American Association of Oriental Medicine: www.aaom.org

American Botanical Counsel—herbal newsletter: www.herbalgram.org

Calorie Restriction Society: www.calorierestriction.org

Canadian College of Naturopathic Medicine: www.ccnm.edu or (866) 241-2266

College Pharmacy—bioidentical hormones in the western U.S.: (800) 888-9358

Daybreak in My Soul—beautiful meditative songs for calm brain balance and for gamma synchrony: www.theforestofpeace.com

DORway—information on artificial sweeteners: www.doorway.com/blayenn.html

Esquimalt Peoples Pharmacy—Alan Hicke, MSc.Pharm, bioidentical hormone replacement compounding specialist in Canada: www.prescriptiondrugsonline.ca

FreshLife Automatic Sprouter—Alpha Health Products: www.alphahealth.ca

Full-spectrum lights, closest light to natural sunlight—Alpha Health Products: www.alphahealth.ca

Genuine Health—free *Health & Happiness* newsletter: www.genuinehealth.com

Glycemic Index (University of Sydney, Australia)—a searchable foods database: www.glycemicindex.com

Grain mills, oat flakers, sprouters, and fermentation crocks—bio supply ltd.: www.biosupply.com

Grass-fed animals—list of farmers: www.eatwild.com and www.pasture-to-plate.com

International Academy of Compounding Pharmacists—natural hormone alternatives to hormone replacement therapy (HRT): (800) 927-4227

International Center for Metabolic Testing—complete blood and hormone testing in Canada: www.icmt.com or (888) 591-4124

Inversion table to lengthen the spinal column and reduce back pain—Green Door Wellness Center: www.greendoorwellness.com

Life Extension Magazine and Life Extension Update: www.lef.org or (800) 544-4440

Meditation CD "Toward Health and Wellness": www.towardstillness.com or (905) 820-4706

National Center for Complementary and Alternative Medicine—supplement information and "searchable" clinical trials: www.nccam.nih.gov

National Institutes of Health (NIH)—great free news on health: www.nih.gov

National Sleep Foundation—sleep information: www.sleepfoundation.org

Nutrition and ORAC information on food: www.nal.usda.gov/fnic/foodcomp/search

Nutritional list of foods and fiber: www.fatfreekitchen.com/fiberlist

Organic food information: www.consumersunion.org

Physicians and Sportsmedicine Online—great information on fitness and nutrition: www.physsportsmed.com

Pilates—Windsor Pilates: www.windsorpilates.com

Qigong—National Qigong Association: www.nqa.org

Tai Chi: www.thetaichisite.com; and www.worldtaichiday.org

USDA Food Pyramid (revised in April 2005): www.mypyramid.gov

Women's Health—National Women's Health Resource Center: www.healthywomen.org

World Health—HealthWorld Online, comprehensive information: www.healthy.net

Wyman, Pat—The Center for New Discoveries in Learning: www.howtolearn.com or (800) 469-8653 for immediate and superior, practical help for all ADD and ADHD conditions

PLEASE NOTE

There are many outstanding osteopathic and chiropractic physicians across North America. A unique, non-invasive approach called the Khan Kinetic Therapy is the most advanced way to realign your skeletal system, joints, and restore neurological circuitry. Dr. Aslam Khan can be reached at www.optimahealthsolutions.com.

References

CHAPTER 1

Barinaga, M. "Life-death within the cell." *Science*, 1996: 274-724.

Cussler, E., T. Lohman et al. "Weight lifted in strength training predicts bone change." *Medicine Science in Sports and Exercise*: 2003, 35:10-17.

Fleming, K.H. et al. "Consumption of calcium in the U.S.: Food sources and intake levels." 1994, *Journal of Nutrition* (8 Suppl): 426-305.

Graci, S. *The Food Connection*. Macmillan, Toronto, 2001.

Myss. C. *Why People Don't Change*. Three Rivers Press, New York, 1997.

National Osteoporosis Foundation. Disease Statistics (Online). Available: http://www.nof.org

Sanson, Gillian. *The Myth of Osteoporosis*. MCD Century Publications, Ann Arbor. 2004.

Starfield, B. "Is US health best in the world?" *The Journal of the American Medical Association, 2000; 284(4): 483-485.*

CHAPTER 2

Dawson-Hughes, B., S. Harris et al. "Effects of calcium and vitamin D supplementation on bone density." *New England Journal of Medicine*, 1997, 323(13): 878-883.

Feskanich, D., P. Weber, W. Willett et al. "Vitamin K intake and hip fractures in women: a prospective study." *American Journal of Clinical Nutrition*, 1999, 69: 74-79.

Graci, S. *The Path to Phenomenal Health*. Wiley & Sons, Toronto, 2005.

Matkovic, V., K. Kostial, I. Simonovic, R. Buzina. "Bone status and fracture rate in two regions of Yugoslavia." *American Journal of Clinical Nutrition*, 1979: 540-549.

Tilgard, M., G. Spears, J. Thompson. "Treatment of osteoporosis with calcitriol or calcium." *New England Journal of Medicine*, 2000, 326(6): 357-362.

Tucker, K., M. Hannon, H. Chen et al. "Potassium, magnesium, fruit and vegetable intakes are associated with greater bone mineral density." *American Journal of Clinical Nutrition*, 1999, 69: 726-736.

Rapp, D. *Is This Your Child?* William Morrow, Quill Books, New York, 1999.

Shils, M., M.D. *Modern Nutrition in Health and Disease,* 8th ed. Lea & Febiger, Philadelphia, 1994.

CHAPTER 3

Bachrach, L.K. "Acquisition of optimal bone mass in childhood and adolescence." *Trends in Endocrionology and Metabolism*, 2001, 12: 22-28.

Graci, S. *The Food Connection*. Macmillan, Toronto, 2001.

Heaney, R.P. "Sources of bone fragility." *Osteoporosis International*, 2000, (Suppl 2): 43-46.

Ott, S., M.D. "Osteoporosis and bone physiology. http://courses.washington.edu/bonephys/

Pors Nielson, S. "The fallacy of BMD: a critical review of the diagnostic use of dual X-ray absorptiometry." *Clinical Rheumatology*, 2000: 174-183.

Polleri, A. et al. "Dementia, a neuroendocrine perspective." *Journal of Endocrinology Investigation*, 2002; 73-83.

Sandyk, R. "Is postmenopausal osteoporosis related to pineal gland functions?" *International Journal of Neuroscience*, 1992: 215-225.

US National Institute of Health (NIH). "Osteoporosis Prevention, Diagnosis and Therapy." Consensus Statement, March, 2000.

CHAPTER 4

Booth, S. "Dietary intake of vitamin K." *Journal of Nutrition*, 1998, 128 (5): 785-788.

Davidson, R. "Conversion of K1 to K2." *Journal of Nutrition*, 1998, 128(2): 220-223.

Demer, L. "Novel mechanism in accelerated vascular calcification." *Current Opinion Hypertens*, 2002, July; 11(4): 437-443.

Graci, S. *The Power of Superfoods*, Prentice Hall, Toronto, 1997.

Miggiano, G. "Vitamin K and diet." *Clinical Trials*, 2005, 156: 41-46.

Plaza, S. "Vitamin K2 in bone metabolism and osteoporosis." *Alternative Medical Review*, 2005, 10(1): 24-35.

Rao, A.V., Agarwal, S. "Sources of lycopene." *Nutritional Research*, 1999, 19: 305-323.

Ryan-Harshman, M."Bone health; New role for vitamin K." *Canadian Family Physician*, 2004, (50): 993-997.

CHAPTER 5

Agren, J.J. "Fish diet, fish oil and docosahexaenoic acid and lipid levels." *European Journal of Clinical Nutrition*, 1996; 50: 765-771.

Ames, B. "Are vitamin and mineral deficiencies a major risk?" *National Review of Cancer*, 2002: 694-704.

Barringer, T. "Effect of a multivitamin and mineral supplement on the quality of life." *Annual International Medicine*, 2003: 365-371.

Earnest, C. "Efficacy of a complex multivitamin supplement." *Nutrition*, 2002: 738-742.

Heaney, R. "Calcium absorption from Kale." *American Journal of Clinical Nutrition*, 1990; 51: 656-660.

CHAPTER 6

Beecher, G. "Phytonutrients' role in metabolism." *Nutrition Reviews*, 1999; 57: 53-56.

Bravo, L. "Polyphenols: chemistry, dietary sources, metabolism and nutritional significance." *Nutrition Reviews*, 1998; 56: 317-333.

Dragland, S. "Several culinary and medicinal herbs are important sources of dietary antioxidants." *Journal of Nutrition*, 2003; 133: 1286-1290.

Elias, M. "Enhancement of natural immune function by dietary consumption of Bifidobacteriium." *European Journal of Clinical Nutrition*, 2000; 54(3): 263-267.

Ferrara, L. et al. "Olive oil and reduced need for antihypertensive medications." *Archives of Internal Medicine*, 2000; 160: 837-842.

Hakkinen, S. et al. "Content of the flavonols in 25 edible berries." *Journal of Agricultural Food Chemistry*, 1999; 47: 2274-2279.

Hu, F. "Fish and omega-3 fatty acid intake and risk of disease." *Journal of the American Medical Association*, 2002; 287: 1815-1821.

Knekt, P. et al. "Flavonoid intake and risk of chronic diseases." *American Journal of Clinical Nutrition*, 2002; 76: 560-568.

Logan, A. *The Brain Diet*. Cumberland House, Nashville, 2006.

Martin, K. et al. "The effect of carotenoids." *Atherosclerosis*, 1999; 150: 265-274.

New, S. et al. "Dietary influences on bone mass and bone metabolism: further evidence of a positive link between fruit and vegetable consumption and bone health." *American Journal of Clinical Nutrition*, 2002; 71: 142-151.

Zimmerman, M. *Eat Your Colors! Maximize Your Health by Eating the Right Foods for Your Body Type*. Henry Holt, New York, 2001.

CHAPTER 7

Brazel, S. "The skeleton as an ion exchange system: implications for the role of acid-base imbalance in the genesis of osteoporosis." *Journal of Bone Mineral Research*, Oct; 10(10): 1431-1436.

Fernando, R. et al. "Consumption of soft drinks with phosphoric acid as a risk factor." 1999, *Journal of Clinical Epidemiology*; 52(10): 1007-1010.

Frassetto, L. et al. "A long-term persistence of the urine calcium-lowering effect of potassium bicarbonate in postmenopausal women." *Journal of Clinical Endocrinology and Metabolism*, Vol. 90. 2005: 831-834.

Graci, S. *The Power of Superfoods*, Prentice Hall, Toronto, 1991.

Graci, S. *The Path to Phenomenal Health*, Wiley & Sons, Toronto, 2005.

Hall, P. "Preventing kidney stones: calcium restriction not warranted." *Cleveland Clinical Journal of Medicine*, 2002; 69(11): 885-888.

Kellum, J. "Determinants of blood pH in health and disease." *Critical Care*, 2000; 4: 6-14.

CHAPTER 8

Graci, S. *The Power of Superfoods*. Prentice Hall, Toronto, 1997

Graci, S. *The Food Connection*. Macmillan, Toronto, 2001

Graci, S. *The Path to Phenomenal Health.* Wiley & Sons, Toronto, 2005.

Zimmerman, M. *Eat Your Colors! Maximize Your Health by Eating the Right Foods for Your Body Type.* Henry Holt, New York, 2001.

CHAPTER 9

Boreham, C. "Training effects of accumulated daily stair-climbing exercises." *Preventive Medicine,* 2000; 30: 277-281.

Dash, M. "Yoga training and motor speed." *Indian Journal of Physiology and Pharmacology,* 1999; 43: 458-462.

Giampapa, V., M.D. *Exercise and Aging.* 2003, Giampapa Institute for Anti-Aging Medicine, Newark, NJ: 2003.

Leipzig, R. et al. "Free and flexible." *Focus on Healthy Aging,* 2002; 5: 4-5.

McCaffery, R. et al. "Qigong practice." *Holistic Nurses Practice,* 2002; 17: 110-116.

Roth, S. et al. "Bone size responds to strength training." *Journal of the American Geriatric Society,* 2001; 49: 1428-1433.

Sinaki, M. et al. "Stronger back muscles reduce the incidence of vertebral fractures." *Bone,* 2002; 30: 836-841.

Springen, K. "Concentrating on the body's core." *Newsweek;* Jan 20, 2003.

CHAPTER 10

Boon, H. et al. "The Effects of *greens+*." *Journal of Dietetic Practice and Research,* August 2004.

Cherniske, S. *The Metabolic Plan.* Ballantine Books, 2003.

Cutler, R.G. "Antioxidants and Aging." *American Journal of Clinical Nutrition,* 1999; Vol. 53: 373-379.

Garland, F. "Sunlight, Vitamin D, and Cancer." *International Journal of Epidemiology,* 1994; Vol. 23: 1133-1136.

Karst, K. *The Metabolic Syndrome Program,* Wiley & Sons, Toronto, 2006.

Natural Medicines Comprehensive Database. www.naturaldatabase.

Rao, V. "The Invitro and Invivo Antioxidant Effects of *greens+*." *Journal of Medicinal Foods,* Fall 2005.

Stevens, L. et al. "Fish Oils ADD/ADHD." *Lipids*, January, 2003.

Vanderhaegh, L.R., and K. Kartst. *Healthy Fats for Life.* Quarry Health Books, Kingston, 2003.

CHAPTER 11

Cosman, Felicia, "The Prevention and Treatment of Osteoporosis: A Review", *Medscape General Medicine* 7(2): 73, 2005

Osteoporosis: Prevention, Diagnosis and Therapy. National Institutes of Health Consensus Development Statement, March 27-29, 2000.

Ott, Susan, http://courses.washington.edu

National Osteoporosis Foundation's Physician's Guide; www.nof.org/phys-guide

Sanson, Gillian, " The Myth of Osteoporosis" 2003, *MCD Century Publications;* http://www.gilliansanson.com

S. Pors Nielsen, "The Fallacy of BMD: A Critical Review of the Diagnostic Use of Dual X-Ray Absorptiometry" *Clin Rheumatol* (2000) 19: 174-183.

Simmons A., et al "Dual Energy X-Ray Absorptiometry Normal Reference Range within the UK and the Effect of Different Normal Ranges on the Assessement of Bone Density" 1995, *The British Journal of Radiology,* 68, 903-909.

Kazanjian A, et al, British Columbia Office of Health Technology Assessment (BCOHTA) "Beyond the Clinical Effectiveness of Bone Mineral Testing in BC: A Comprehensive Approach to Health Technology Assessment." *BCOHTA*: 00:5C, April 2000.

Ibid. "Normal Bone Mass, Aging Bodies, Marketing of Fear: Bone Mineral Density Screening of Well Women." *BCOHTA* 98:10C September 1998

Ibid. "Bone Mineral Density; Does the Evidence Support Its Selective Use in Well Women?" *BCOHTA* 97:2T December 1997

BC Health Services: Guidelines and Protocols for Bone Density Measurement in Women, Revised 2005.

Gurlek A, et al, "Inappropriate Reference Ranges for Peak Bone Mineral Density in Dual-energy X-Ray Absorptiometry; Implications for the Interpretation of T-scores." *Osteoporosis* (2000) 11, 809-813.

Ahmed, A.I. H. et al, "Screening for Osteopenia and Osteoporosis: Do the Accepted Normal Ranges Lead to Overdiagnosis?" *Osteoporosis International* (1997) 7: 432-438.

CHAPTER 12

Harris, Steven T. " New Considerations in the Selection of Current Therapies to Prevent and Treat Osteoporosis." *Medscape CME* December 30, 2002.

Dennis Black et al, "Fracture Risk Reduction with Alendronate in Women With Osteoporosis: The Fracture Intervention Trial" *The Journal of Clinical Endocrinology and Metabolism,* Vol 85 (11) 4118-4124.

Hodsman A.B. "Parathyroid Hormone and Teriparatide for the Treatment of Osteoporosis: A Review of the Evidence and Suggested Guidelines for Use" *Endocrine Reviews* 26(5) 688-703.

Cranney Ann, Adachi, Jonathan, "Benefit Risk Assessment of Raloxifene in Postmenopausal Osteoporosis." *Drug Safety* 2005; 288 (8) 721-30.

Farrugia MC, et al, "Osteonecrosis of the mandible or maxilla associated with the use of new generation bisphosphonates." *Laryngoscope* 2006; 116 (1) 115-20

CHAPTER 13

1. Lindsay, R., Cosman, F. 1999. In: Favus, M.J. (ed.) *Primer on the Metabolic Bone Diseases and Disorders of Mineral Metabolism.* New York: Lippincott Williams & Wilkins, pp. 264–270.

2. Consensus Development Conference. 1993. *American Journal of Medicine* 94:646–650.

3. Raisz, L.G. 2005. *Journal of Clinical Investigation* 115(12):3318–3325.

4. Pietschmann, P., Kerschan-Schindl, K. 2004. *Wiener Medizinische Wochenschrift* 154(17–18):411–415.

5. Garnero, P., Sornay-Rendu, E., Chapuy, M.-C., Delmas, P.D. 1996. *Journal Bone Mineral Research* 11(3):337–349.

6. Srivastava, A.K., Vliet, E.L., Lewiecki, E.M., et al. 2005. *Current Medical Research & Opinion* 21(7):1015–1026.

7. Urquiaga, I., Leighton, F. 2000. *Biological Research* 33:55–64.

8. Hegarty, V.M., Helen, M.M., Khaw, K. 2000. *American Journal of Clinical Nutrition* 71:1003–1007.

9. Yun, J.H., Pang, E.K., Kim, C.S., et al. 2004 *Journal of Periodontal Research* 39(5):300–307.

10. Park, Y.H., Han, D.W., Suh, H., et al. 2003. *Cell Biology & Toxicology* 19(5):325–337.

11. Puel, C., Quintin, A., Mathey, J., et al. 2005 *Calcified Tissue International* 77(5):311–318.

12. Balachandran, B., Rao, A.V., Murray, T., Rao, L.G. 2004. Presented to the 27th Annual Meeting of the American Society of Bone and Mineral research, Nashville, TN, 2005, Seattle, Washington.

13. Rao, L.G., Balachandran, B., Rao, A.V. 2005. Presented to the 27th Annual Meeting of the American Society of Bone and Mineral research, Nashville, TN, September 23–27.

14. Rao, A.V., Agarwal, S. 1999. *Nutrition Research* 19:305–323.

15. Clinton, S.K. 1998. *Nutrition Reviews* 1:35–51.

16. Zhang, L.X., Cooney, R.V., Bertram, J.S. 1991. Carcinogenesis 12:2109–2114.

17. Amir, H., Karas, M., Giat, J., Danilenko, M., et al. 1999 *Nutrition & Cancer* 33:105–112.

18. Rao, A.V., Shen, H.L. 2002. *Nutrition Research*:1125–1131.

19. Rao, L.G., Krishnadev, N., Banasikowska, K., Rao, A.V. 2003. *Journal of Medicinal Food* 6(2):69–78.

20. Ishimi, Y., Ohmura, M., Wang, X., et al. 1999 *Journal of Clinical Biochemical Nutrition* 27:113–122.

21. Park, C.K., Ishimi, Y., Ohmura, M., et al. 1997 *Journal of Nutritional Science & Vitaminology* 43:281–296.

22. Kim, L., Rao, A.V., Rao, L.G. 2003. *Journal of Medicinal Food* 6(2):79–86.

23. Rao, L.G., Collins, E.S., Josse, R.G., et al. 2005 Joint Meeting of the ECTS and IBMS Geneva, Switzerland, June 25–29.

24. Vernejoul, M.-C. de. 1998. *Drugs & Aging* 1 (supplement 1):9–14.

25. Kushida, K., Takahashi, M., Kawana, K., Inoue, T. 1995. *Journal of Clinical Endocrinology Metabolism* 80(8):2447–2450.

Index